The
Thyroid
Guide

D0029214

The
Thyroid
Guide

**Beth Ann Ditkoff, M.D. ,
and Paul Lo Gerfo, M.D.**

HarperPerennial
An Imprint of HarperCollins*Publishers*

THIS BOOK IS NOT INTENDED TO REPLACE MEDICAL ADVICE OR BE A SUBSTITUTE FOR A PHYSCIAN. ALWAYS SEEK THE ADVICE OF A PHYSICIAN.

THE THYROID GUIDE. Copyright © 2000 by Beth Ann Ditkoff, M.D., and Paul Lo Gerfo, M.D. All rights reserved. Printed in the United States of America. No part of this book may be used or reproduced in any manner whatsoever without written permission except in the case of brief quotations embodied in critical articles and reviews. For information address HarperCollins Publishers Inc., 10 East 53rd Street, New York, NY 10022.

HarperCollins books may be purchased for educational, business, or sales promotional use. For information please write: Special Markets Department, HarperCollins Publishers Inc., 10 East 53rd Street, New York, NY 10022.

FIRST EDITION

Printer on acid-free paper

Designed by Liane F. Fuji

Library of Congress Cataloging-in-Publication Data

Ditkoff, Beth Ann.
    The thyroid guide/Beth Ann Ditkoff and Paul Lo Gerfo.—1st ed.
        p.   cm.
    ISBN 0-06-095260-1
        1. Thyroid gland—Diseases Popular works.   I. Lo Gerfo, Paul.
    II. Title
    RC655.D58   2000
    616.4'4—dc21   99–34742

00 01 02 03 04 ❖/RRD 10 9 8 7 6 5 4 3 2 1

To SLBZ
—BD

My parents,
Phillis and Paul Lo Gerfo
—PL

Contents

Introduction and Overview of the Thyroid

For more than twenty years, a group of physicians at the Columbia Presbyterian Medical Center in New York City have met every Friday morning at nine-thirty to discuss the care and treatment of patients with thyroid disease. In 1995, these physicians formalized their interest and created the Thyroid Center. A vast array of physicians joined this group. Some were medical doctors, endocrinologists, who were concerned with diagnosing and treating thyroid disease with medications. Thyroid surgeons identified patients with thyroid cancer and performed operations to help cure the disease. Thyroid pathologists looked at the thyroid gland underneath the microscope to help sort out the many different types of thyroid disorders. Ophthalmologists were dedicated to treating the troublesome eye problems that can result from some types of thyroid disease. Radiologists were interested in special X-ray tests to help better identify patients with thyroid lumps that may be cancerous. All of these physicians got together because of their intense interest in learning more about thyroid disease, to pool their knowledge and to promote a more unified, efficient, and compassionate way to care for patients with thyroid disorders.

A few years ago, as a member of the Thyroid Center, I was asked to give a lecture to a group of patients with thyroid disease. The title of my talk was "Everything You Always Wanted to Know About Thyroid Disease But Were Afraid to Ask Your Doctor." The topic is enormous, and I was expected to address all of the different types of thyroid disease—underactive and overactive thyroid illnesses, lumps in the thyroid, children with thyroid disease, and thyroid illness during and after pregnancy. All of this in only sixty minutes! Condensing this information was a daunting task, but the biggest challenge was getting over my fear of addressing an audience of potentially bored and confused patients. How much did these patients really want to know?

To my relief, the lecture was extremely well received. I discovered that because thyroid illnesses are lifelong conditions, many thyroid patients are hungry for details about the disease and information on treatment options. In response to the patients' demand for more information than I could provide in one hour, my colleagues and I began to write down everything we know.

We drafted pamphlets for our office practice describing the fatigue and weight gain associated with hypothyroidism (an underactive thyroid). We wrote about hyperthyroidism (overactive thyroid) and the nervousness and insomnia seen with this illness. We wrote a separate pamphlet on thyroid nodules or lumps, which affect 5 percent of the world's population. With each pamphlet that we wrote explaining thyroid disease, we received more and more positive feedback from our patients, who are intensely interested in understanding their illness. It soon became clear that a full-length book was in order.

Thyroid disease is extremely common in the United States. In fact, over 20 million people are currently receiving treatment for thyroid disorders. An estimated 2 million others have an undiagnosed thyroid problem. The majority of thyroid disease affects women, although we don't really understand why it affects women more often than men.

Despite the prevalence of thyroid disease, thyroid disorders are often undiagnosed because the symptoms are usually subtle. Both you and your doctor may have a hard time even noticing these symptoms if they appear slowly and over many months or years. For example, a patient with an underactive thyroid, a condition called hypothyroidism, may have symptoms of fatigue, weight gain, and loss of energy. A patient with an overactive thyroid may complain of nervousness or difficulty sleeping at night. Since these complaints are common, many patients and doctors overlook these relatively innocuous symptoms and do not make the diagnosis of thyroid disease. Caroline is an example:

I'm a forty-five-year-old woman with three children and a full-time career as an attorney. Over the past several years, I have felt more and more tired and run down. I've gained fifteen pounds even though I keep trying to diet. Lately, I've been feeling depressed and down in the dumps. I'm always arguing with my husband and I have absolutely zero interest in sex. When I look in the mirror, a tired, puffy-eyed face looks back at me.

I told my gynecologist about these symptoms and he told me I was just working too hard. I told my internist about my problems and she said—"What do you expect with a full-time career, a husband, and three children?"

At first I just believed them—I mean, after all, I'm not

twenty years old anymore. Maybe I'm just working too hard. But even last year I felt I had more energy than this. Something must be wrong. I used to be a vibrant woman. Now, I'm blue all the time and find it difficult to concentrate on anything.

Finally, Caroline saw a third doctor who tested her for thyroid disease, made the diagnosis of an underactive thyroid, and started Caroline on the medication that she needed to have normal thyroid function.

Eight weeks later (when the medicine reached its full effect) Caroline felt like her old self again. Her doctor is continuing to monitor her condition with yearly office visits and blood tests.

We dedicate this book to the millions of Americans with thyroid disease in order that they may better understand the symptoms, diagnosis, and treatment options for their illness. We hope that our book educates patients and families about all aspects of thyroid disease. When patients are given the opportunity to understand their illness, they can successfully participate in their treatment.

Finding Your Thyroid Gland

The thyroid gland is located in the front of the neck and on top of the windpipe or trachea. It is also near the swallowing tube, the esophagus. Because the gland is in the front of the throat, it is often easy to see abnormal enlargement or lumps that can be the first sign of thyroid disease. A very enlarged thyroid gland may press on the trachea or esophagus, causing difficulty breathing or difficulty swallowing solid foods.

The American Association of Clinical Endocrinologists, as

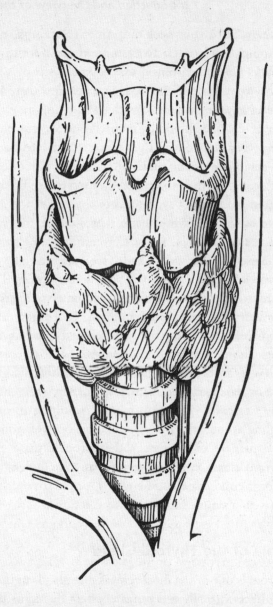

Human Throat with Larynx, Thyroid, Carotid Artery,
Esophagus, Trachea exposed

part of their "Stick your neck out, America" campaign, recommends a quick "neck check" to examine yourself for thyroid disease. While holding a mirror, take a small sip of water and watch the front of your throat as you swallow. Any lumps or bumps in this area that move with swallowing may represent thyroid nodules and should be pointed out to your physician.

The nerves that control the voice box are located near the thyroid gland. So some patients with thyroid disease may notice changes in their voice if these nerves are affected. For instance, one of the first symptoms of thyroid cancer may be a hoarse voice if the thyroid cancer presses on the voice-box nerves. The thyroid is also in close proximity to the parathyroid glands. These are four tiny glands (two on the right side and two on the left) that control the body's calcium level. If these glands are overactive as a result of a benign or rarely malignant tumor your calcium level may be high. Too much calcium in the bloodstream can cause many different types of symptoms, including kidney stones, osteoporosis, or even psychiatric changes (such as mood swings). If these parathyroid glands are removed or damaged during thyroid surgery (see chapter 6), the body's calcium may drop rapidly, resulting in numbness and tingling around the mouth, seizures, or even coma. Since about 10 percent of patients with thyroid disease also have parathyroid disease, it is important for anyone undergoing evaluation for thyroid disease to be tested for parathyroid function as well (with a simple blood test for calcium).

The Role of the Thyroid Gland

The thyroid is one of the most remarkable glands in the human body. It affects virtually every organ system including the brain, heart, intestines, skin, and so many others. Thyroid hormone, produced by the thyroid, acts as the electricity that keeps the busy factory—your body—running efficiently and smoothly. The thyroid gland is like an energy source for a small factory. Without power and electricity, the machines in the factory cannot operate. The building becomes cold. The windows become coated with frost. No products can be produced by the factory, and eventually all work comes to a grinding halt. The thyroid gland provides this same energy and power source for your body. Every organ system is affected by the fuel, or thyroid hormone. Without this thyroid hormone, the body's metabolism slows and the body begins to feel sluggish. It becomes difficult to concentrate. The body begins to gain weight. The skin is cold and dry. All of these symptoms are a direct result of not having enough thyroid hormone.

Although the thyroid and some of its disorders were described hundreds of years ago, it is only during the last one hundred years that we have been able to accurately characterize the exact anatomy of the thyroid gland as well as the role of thyroid hormone. Long ago, physicians believed that the job of the thyroid was to fill out the hollow portions of a woman's neck in order to make it more round and beautiful. Others hypothesized that the thyroid gland was a hernia of the windpipe. Finally, others thought that the thyroid was filled with worms that aided in digestion.

Because doctors did not know what the thyroid did, they thought that it was not a necessary organ—just as we believe that the appendix has no definite role in maintaining a healthy body. Although they did not know the function of the thyroid, physicians knew that the thyroid gland could sometimes enlarge, called a goiter. If this goiter became very large, it could slowly encircle the windpipe over many years until the patient suffocated to death. Despite knowing about goiter, surgery to remove the thyroid was virtually unheard of before the late nineteenth century. Prior to that time, operations on the thyroid were usually lethal because of overwhelming bleeding or infection. In more modern times, with the use of sterile technique and more accurate surgery to avoid bleeding, thyroid surgery gradually became more successful.

However, in following these early patients who underwent thyroid surgery, it was noted that over time, they became progressively obese and intellectually impaired. Eventually, they lapsed into coma. Children undergoing thyroid surgery experienced stunted growth and mental retardation. These observations led to the discovery of thyroid hormone's essential role in the body's normal growth and function. Theodor Kocher, one of the earliest thyroid surgeons, received the Nobel prize in medicine in 1909 for this important discovery.

It was later noted that people in iodine deficient areas of the country (remember that iodine is found in salt, so people who lived inland—in the Midwest, for example—who did not have access to saltwater oceans and saltwater fish were iodine deficient) developed thyroid enlargement or goiter. Iodine is an essential nutrient for the body, particularly for the thyroid. Without iodine, the thyroid cannot produce thyroid hormone. With the routine addition of iodine in the diet (by iodinizing the salt), this type of diet-related, or *endemic*, goiter has been virtually eliminated in the United States and most developed countries. There are other causes of goiter besides iodine deficiency and these are reviewed in chapter 4.

More recently, we have found that the thyroid helps to control the body's metabolism by supplying energy to virtually every organ system in the body. Too much thyroid hormone, or *hyperthyroidism*, speeds up the metabolism. So, for example, a patient with hyperthyroidism may experience symptoms of a racing heart, excessive perspiration, and anxiety. Too little thyroid hormone, or *hypothyroidism*, may cause the symptoms of weight gain, constipation, dry skin, and depression. Many of the symptoms of hyperthyroidism such as weight loss, decreased appetite, racing heartbeat, and nervousness are also symptoms that can be seen in pregnancy. (At the beginning of this century, special "clinics" were set up for young women with overactive thyroids. These were, in fact, illegal abortion houses that claimed to treat thyroid disease.)

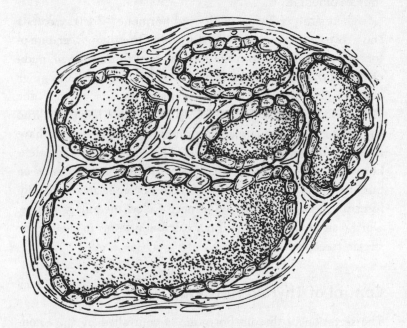

Thyroid Follicle Cells with Colloid

When you look at the thyroid gland underneath a microscope it looks like a field with many lakes. The water in the lake is called *colloid*. Each lake is called a *follicle*. Each follicle is lined by a fence. Each picket of the fence is a thyroid follicular cell. These are the cells that are responsible for producing thyroid hormone.

Thyroglobulin, a special protein produced exclusively by the thyroid cell, sits in the center of the lake. Thyroglobulin is the protein used in combination with iodine to form thyroid hormone. As noted above, the body gets its iodine from foods that we eat. In the United States, iodine is routinely added to salt, so any foods that contain iodized salt are a good source of iodine. In addition, saltwater fish and seafood are also excellent sources of iodine.

There are two forms of thyroid hormone—T4 (thyroxine) and T3 (triiodothyronine). T4 is made in the thyroid, and once formed, it is released into the bloodstream to travel to all parts of the body. In the bloodstream, T4 is converted to T3 in other organs such as the liver, muscles, and kidneys.

In addition to the thyroid follicular cells that line the colloid lakes of the thyroid, there are also thyroid cells in between these lakes called *parafollicular* or C cells. These special cells secrete a hormone called *calcitonin*. No one truly knows its function or purpose in humans, but if these C cells become cancerous, they form a rare type of thyroid cancer called medullary cancer, which can be diagnosed by high calcitonin levels in the bloodstream (see chapter 5).

Control of Thyroid Hormone

The secretion of thyroid hormone is controlled by the brain. First, thyrotropin releasing hormone (TRH) is produced by the hypothalamus portion of the brain, which then sends a positive message to another part of the brain called the pituitary gland. Here, thyroid-stimulating hormone (TSH) is produced, which does exactly what its name implies, stimulates the thyroid to release thyroid hormone.

An elaborate feedback mechanism controls the level of thyroid hormone in the bloodstream. For example, if there is too much thyroid hormone in the bloodstream, a negative message is sent to the brain, which turns down the secretion of TRH and TSH, thus causing less thyroid hormone to be released from the thyroid gland. The opposite is also true: if there is not enough thyroid hormone in the bloodstream, the brain is stimulated to produce more TRH and thus, in turn, more TSH to increase thyroid hormone production by the thyroid gland.

If either the hypothalamus or pituitary gland is malfunctioning as a result of trauma or a brain tumor, this delicate balance between TRH and TSH can be upset, resulting in the wrong amount of thyroid hormone production.

All in the Family

Thyroid disease commonly runs in families. In addition, you can be at risk if you have a medical history or someone in your family has a history of autoimmune disease, a disorder of your body's immune system. Something happens to the immune system, so that instead of fighting off attacks on your body (like from bacteria that cause infection), the immune system attacks your own body. For example, in diabetes, your body's immune system attacks the part of your pancreas that makes insulin, causing high sugar levels in the bloodstream. Other examples of autoimmune diseases include vitiligo (a disease that results in areas of skin that lose their color), rheumatoid arthritis, pernicious anemia, or prematurely graying hair. These diseases can lead to the development of autoimmune thyroid diseases such as Graves' disease or Hashimoto's thyroiditis.

In addition, some types of thyroid cancer may be inherited. Medullary thyroid cancer often runs in families, and about 5 percent of all papillary thyroid cancers are hereditary (see also chapter 5).

Life Without Your Thyroid Gland

You can live without your thyroid gland. If the thyroid is surgically removed or destroyed as a result of disease, thyroid hormone medication will be given for the rest of your life. When placed on the correct dose of thyroid hormone medication, you will not experience any consequences of your missing thyroid gland (see Appendix II for more information on thyroid hormone medications).

1

Choosing Your Thyroid Physician

Choosing a physician for any medical problem is not easy, and finding one who is skilled in thyroid disorders can be particularly difficult. Because thyroid diseases are usually lifelong, thyroid patients require not only an experienced physician, but one who is able to develop a respectful and long-term relationship with their patients.

For medical thyroid problems (such as an under- or overactive thyroid), that is, those that do not require operation, a patient should choose a medical doctor (as opposed to a surgeon). Your choice may include an internist, a family practice physician, or a medical endocrinologist, a specialist who is trained in a variety of endocrine diseases (hormone disorders) such as thyroid and parathyroid disease as well as diabetes and other hormonal ailments.

If you require radioactive iodine to treat thyroid cancer you will be referred to a radiologist who specializes in nuclear medicine.

If your thyroid disease requires an operation you will have

to choose a surgeon. Many different types of surgeons perform thyroid operations, including general surgeons, head and neck surgeons (also sometimes called ENT surgeons for ear, nose, and throat, or otorhinolaryngolosists), or even plastic surgeons. All of these surgeons may be trained to perform thyroid surgery, but the real difference lies in their experience with this type of operation. For example, although an ENT surgeon is very comfortable doing operations of the throat, he may not perform many thyroid operations in the course of a year. This may mean that he has little experience with thyroid disease and be unfamiliar recognizing thyroid abnormalities during an operation. Don't be afraid to ask how many thyroid operations your surgeon performs every year (see below).

If you need a special test such as an ultrasound, computerized tomography scan (CT scan), or nuclear scan, a radiologist will read and interpret the test.

Regardless of what type of thyroid ailment you have, it is still critical to thoroughly screen your physician to make sure that you are getting the best care. Below are some important questions for you to consider.

How well trained is your thyroid doctor?

Where did your doctor go to medical school and where did he do his residency or training after medical school? If your doctor trained outside the country, has he been certified to practice this specialty in the United States?

Has your doctor done specialized training in thyroid disease? For example, a qualified internist may have done an additional fellowship in medical endocrinology, which includes thyroid disease. An appropriate surgeon may have trained in thyroid and parathyroid surgery by doing an additional fellowship in endocrine surgery in addition to his or her previous training.

Is your physician board certified in his or her field? Has your doctor passed strict written and/or oral examinations in his or her area of expertise?

Does your doctor have experience treating patients with thyroid disease?

It is important to ask your doctor what percentage of his or her practice is devoted to thyroid disease. For medical physicians and radiologists the answer to this question should be at least 25 percent. There are some medical endocrinologists, for example, who although originally trained to treat patients with thyroid disease, rarely in fact see patients with thyroid disorders. Obviously, these would not be the ideal doctors for you.

For a thyroid surgeon, ask what part of his practice involves thyroid/parathyroid surgery. Remember that there are risks to thyroid surgery (see chapter 7) and although these complications can never be eliminated entirely, they can be minimized in the hands of an experienced thyroid surgeon. Your surgeon should perform at least twenty-five thyroid and/or parathyroid operations per year. If your surgeon performs less than that number, look for a different surgeon.

Again, remember that just because someone is trained in head and neck surgery doesn't necessarily mean that he or she is skilled in performing thyroid operations. Because much of the decision-making process regarding the extent of thyroid surgery and the type of operation performed depends on your physician's judgment during your operation, it is important to have a surgeon with a lot of thyroid experience.

You should also ask your thyroid surgeon how many of the thyroid operations that he performs are for cancer. This number is important, because, as we discuss in the section on thyroid lumps or nodules, there are many instances where a thyroid operation is the only way to tell if a patient has thyroid cancer or not. The preoperative tests to diagnose thyroid cancer are limited, but still effective. At least 25 percent of the patients undergoing thyroid surgery should have either precancer or cancer. A figure lower than this one, means that your thyroid surgeon is not screening patients preoperatively and may be performing unnecessary operations. Some hospitals have a rate as low as 10 percent, while other major thyroid centers may have a figure as high as 50 percent.

Academic Activities

It's a good idea to find a doctor who is affiliated with a thyroid center—a multidisciplinary group of physicians and practitioners designed to diagnose, treat, and educate patients with thyroid disease. A thyroid center has radiologists, pathologists, ophthalmologists, medical endocrinologists, endocrine surgeons, and other practitioners who focus their practice on the treatment of thyroid disease.

Additionally, you should ask if your practitioner has any affiliations with national academic societies specifically concerning thyroid disease, such as the American Thyroid Association, the Endocrine Society, the American Association of Clinical Endocrinologists (for medical doctors), the American Association of Endocrine Surgeons, the Society of Head and Neck Surgeons (for surgeons).

Remember to ask questions about academic activities—

does your thyroid surgeon do any thyroid research—either clinical or basic science? If the answer is yes, you know that your doctor has a significant career interest in thyroid disorders.

Never be afraid to ask these questions in order to provide yourself with the physician who is best for your particular problem. Remember that the field of thyroid disease is an area of intense academic interest with new research developments constantly being discovered. You want a physician who is abreast of this current research and can provide you with the latest in treatment in addition to educating you about your thyroid disorder.

Are there any holistic practitioners or complementary care alternatives I can pursue?

Although alternative medical approaches can alleviate many of the symptoms of chronic thyroid disorders, none has ever been proven to cure these illnesses. Some academic medical centers are affiliated with complementary care centers. Ask your doctor for a referral. If you choose a complementary care doctor instead of a conventional physician, we would advise that you talk to other patients who have tried a similar approach with the same doctor or practitioner.

Remember that any herbal medicines or vitamins prescribed must be evaluated with the help of your physician to avoid the inadvertent taking of substances that may worsen your condition. For example, excessive doses of iodine found in sea kelp tablets may worsen the symptoms of hyperthyroidism (see chapter 9).

It is so hard to find a specialist—can't I just use my family physician to treat my thyroid illness?

Recent studies have shown that it is much more efficient and cost effective to go to a medical endocrinologist rather than a family doctor if you have a thyroid lump. Twenty-five percent of patients who were referred by their family doctor to an endocrinologist for evaluation of a thyroid nodule didn't even have any nodule when they were examined by an experienced thyroid doctor. Further, the diagnostic tests ordered by the medical endocrinologist were much less costly and more efficient than those tests ordered by their family doctor. These studies only focused on patients with thyroid lumps, not other illnesses such as an overactive or underactive thyroid, but the same principle applies. Thyroid illnesses should be treated by physicians who see and treat thyroid problems on a regular basis, not just once in a while (see above).

Is my doctor right for me?

Once you've found a thyroid doctor, it's time to ask the question, "Is this doctor right for me?" You've already done all your homework regarding his thyroid credentials, now you want to know if your doctor has the right personality and "bedside manner" for you. Are you given the opportunity to ask questions, or do you feel rushed and hurried at your office visits? Does your doctor or the doctor's staff call or write promptly to let you know the results of recent tests? Does your doctor seem to know your medical history? Are explanations clear or are they just medical jargon? Take the time to find a doctor that matches your personality. Remember that most thyroid illnesses are lifelong, so it's worthwhile finding a doctor with whom you can form a long-term relationship.

For more help in choosing your thyroid physician here are some resources:

The Thyroid Society for Education and Research
7515 South Main Street
Suite 545
Houston, Texas 77030
www.the-thyroid-society.org

This society is a national, not-for-profit group whose mission is "to pursue the prevention, treatment, and cure of thyroid disease." The society provides a series of educational pamphlets specifically designed for people with thyroid disease. These booklets are concise and well written.

The Thyroid Foundation of America, Inc.
Ruth Sleeper Hall, RSL 350
40 Parkman Street
Boston, Massachusetts 02114–2698
www.tfaweb.org/pub/tfa

This is an organization devoted to education and medical referrals. They provide educational brochures and newsletters as well as a toll-free number for referrals of thyroid specialists near your home.

National Graves' Disease Foundation
2 Tsitsi Court
Brevard, North Carolina 28712

A nonprofit organization designed to provide education, information, and support for patients with Graves' disease.

Thyroid e-mailing lists that provide helpful information include:

1. ThyCa (majordomo@world.std.com): This is primarily for thyroid surgery patients who have thyroid cancer.
2. Thyroid (listserv@maelstrom.stjohns.edu): This list provides useful information for people who suffer from chronic thyroid disorders.
3. Thyroid-Onc (listserv@acor.org): This includes information for both thyroid cancer patients and those with benign thyroid diseases.

2
Hypothyroidism

Hypothyroidism is the result of an underactive thyroid gland that doesn't produce enough thyroid hormone. Remember that thyroid hormone is the fuel that drives your body and keeps up your energy level. Without this fuel, your body becomes tired and rundown. Every organ system slows—the brain slows down and it may become difficult to concentrate. You intestines slow down and constipation sets in. Your metabolism slows down and your body begins to gain weight. Although there are many different causes for an underactive thyroid gland, the resulting effect on your body is the same.

Many of the symptoms of hypothyroidism are very subtle and are experienced by people without thyroid disease. Thus, a lot of physicians overlook the symptoms of fatigue, weight gain, and depression and attribute them to other causes. Physicians should check to see if thyroid disease is the cause of these everyday symptoms, because an underactive thyroid is very easy to treat. In addition, patients who are treated for hypothyroidism can regain full control of their lives and eliminate these symptoms entirely.

Who Is at Risk?

The most common cause of hypothyroidism in the United States is a form of thyroid disease called Hashimoto's thyroiditis. The suffix -*itis* means inflammation; just like appendicitis is inflammation of the appendix, thyroiditis is inflammation of the thyroid. This inflammation is caused by an abnormal reaction of the body's immune system. In other words, immune cells that usually fight off infection and colds, suddenly get confused and attack the body itself. In thyroiditis, this attack is directed specifically against the thyroid gland, which slowly becomes destroyed. This type of attack is called an autoimmune disease.

If you have other autoimmune diseases, you may also be at risk for Hashimoto's thyroiditis. Some common examples of these autoimmune diseases include rheumatoid arthritis (the immune cells attack the joints) and diabetes (the immune cells attack the pancreas, which produces insulin). Still other examples of autoimmune diseases include vitiligo (a skin condition in which patches of skin lose their color and become white— Michael Jackson recently told the press that he suffers from this disorder), Addison's disease (President John F. Kennedy suffered from this disorder of the adrenal glands), and pernicious anemia (a special form of low blood count). In fact, about 10 percent of patients with Type I or juvenile diabetes mellitus develop chronic thyroiditis during their life. If you are a diabetic with thyroid disease, the amount of insulin you need every day may change. It is therefore important for diabetic patients to be checked for thyroid disease by routine thyroid function blood tests on a regular basis.

You may be at risk for an underactive thyroid if you are taking a prescription medication that has been shown to cause thyroid disease. For example, if you have a psychiatric disease called manic depressive disorder and are being treated with the drug lithium, you may be at risk. This drug can cause thyroid enlargement and an underproduction of thyroid hormone, resulting in an underactive thyroid.

Here are some examples of the symptoms caused by hypothyroidism:

Feeling Tired

Joe is a twenty-five-year-old student. He has been studying extremely hard for midterm exams and is both overwhelmed and exhausted. Even before midterms began, he started feeling very tired and unmotivated.

> *I am so tired all of the time. When I wake up in the morning I feel exhausted. It's like I just can't catch up. I fall asleep every night studying at my desk. Even when I get a full night's sleep I still feel like I need to put my head on my desk during class. Maybe the stress is just getting to me.*

One of the main symptoms of hypothyroidism is fatigue. Because fatigue has many other causes besides hypothyroidism, it's often overlooked until it becomes severe. Also, the fatigue may start out gradually and only slowly progress to a more extreme form. Many practitioners dismiss patients' complaints of fatigue because they are too vague and nonspecific. But fatigue is a real symptom of hypothyroidism and one that can be easily treated.

Trouble Concentrating

Molly is a fifty-five-year-old housewife. Her youngest child just left for college and she's been feeling very lonely. Her friends tell her that she's just experiencing "empty nest syndrome," but she feels it's more than that. She feels restless and has trouble concentrating. When she goes to the grocery store, even if it's for just a few items, she often forgets something and has to go back.

> Lately I can't seem to concentrate on anything. My memory seems like it's not working right. When I try to read the paper or even watch TV, my mind wanders. What's wrong with me?

This inability to concentrate is classic for hypothyroidism. Again, the symptoms of memory loss and difficulty focusing are very general symptoms that may occur from a variety of causes, not just thyroid disease. Since many people with underactive thyroids are over the age of fifty, they feel that this memory loss is normal, part of the aging process. But, if these symptoms are due to hypothyroidism, they are easily treated and reversed.

Singing the Blues

Sarah is a twenty-five-year-old secretary. She recently split with Jim, her boyfriend of three years, and has been very depressed about the breakup. Sarah had recognized their problems for many months, but she was unable to do anything about them. Jim was always complaining that she was so negative all the time. He would want to go out to parties and have fun, but Sarah just didn't feel like socializing. Her constant bad moods eventually caused their breakup.

> Recently, I've been feeling very down. I just don't feel good about myself anymore. I've been gaining weight and I've

had trouble falling asleep. I'm stressed about my job and
things just don't seem to be working well for me.

Low self-esteem, feelings of unworthiness, weight gain, and sleep disturbances are all symptoms of depression. Although there may be many different causes of depression, one cause may be an underactive thyroid gland or hypothyroidism. Tell your doctor that you are having these feelings. Don't be embarrassed or ashamed. Hypothyroidism is easy to treat.

Crabby, Cranky, and Cantankerous

Victoria is a forty-year-old mother of three who works part time in a law office. Recently she's been feeling very irritable—at work, at home, and with her friends.

I feel nervous and anxious all the time. My husband says
I'm too touchy and we seem to be fighting a lot—not just
about the usual things like finances, but about everything!
I'm short-tempered with my children, even when I don't
mean to be. Yesterday Tommy asked me to help him with
his homework and I nearly bit his head off.
   I just feel like something is wrong—like something
bad is going to happen to me or to my family.

Classically, we associate the symptoms of restlessness, anxiety, irritability, and a sense of "impending doom" with an overactive thyroid or hyperthyroidism. However, sometimes the symptoms of hyperthyroidism and hypothyroidism may in fact overlap. The symptoms may be vague and often you just don't feel like yourself. You can't quite put your finger on the problem, but you know that something is wrong.

There's No Diet I Haven't Tried . . .

Samantha is a forty-two-year-old bank teller who has been trying to lose weight for over two years. After her first child was born, she had no problem losing the extra weight in just a few months. But after her second child was born, she never took the weight off. In fact, she just kept putting on the pounds.

> *I keep on gaining weight no matter what I do. I've tried every diet. I even joined a gym, but I just keep gaining weight. What's the matter with me?*

There are many causes of weight gain and obesity. Hypothyroidism is just one cause. If you don't produce enough thyroid hormone, you have a slower metabolism and therefore tend to gain weight, despite dieting and cutting calories. Although hypothyroidism is not the most common cause of being overweight in this country, it is certainly an easily treatable and reversible one.

Infertility

Amanda and Jim are both twenty-seven years old. They have been married for three years.

> *My husband and I have been trying to become pregnant. We've been trying for over a year now, but still haven't been successful. My periods are not regular and sometimes I don't even get them at all. Every time I miss a cycle we get excited and think that this is it. But the pregnancy test always turns up negative. We are thinking about going to see an infertility specialist.*

An important part in the initial work-up of any woman who is having trouble getting pregnant is basic thyroid blood tests. An underactive thyroid gland may lead to irregular ovulation and irregular periods (which at times can be quite heavy) thus making it difficult to become pregnant. Although infertility usually only occurs in severe cases of hypothyroidism, even mild cases may contribute to these irregular cycles.

Feeling Cold

Enid is a sixty-five-year-old retired schoolteacher.

> *I feel cold all the time. Even in the summer when the weather is hot, I'm never comfortable. My husband is always turning on the air conditioner and I'm turning it off.*

Feeling cold when other people feel comfortable is a common symptom of hypothyroidism, just as feeling hot and sweaty when other people feel comfortable is a symptom associated with hyperthyroidism. People with hypothyroidism feel chilly, even when other people in the room feel the room temperature is comfortable.

Thinning Hair

Catherine is an eighteen-year-old college student.

> *My skin has become so dry. I use cream on my legs, but they are always so flaky. My nails keep on breaking and my hair is falling out in little clumps. What's the matter with me?*

Again, an underactive thyroid can cause all of these symptoms including dry skin, a puffy face (especially under the eyelids), brittle nails, loss of eyebrow hair (on the outsides), and thinning hair.

Getting Older

Maria is concerned about her elderly mother who lives on her own in an apartment nearby.

> *My mother is eighty-five years old and she's really having a lot of problems. She's unsteady on her feet and she feels weak. Lately, she's been having a lot of trouble with constipation. The doctor told us that it's all part of the aging process—as you age everything slows down. But, it just doesn't seem right.*

Many of the changes that occur with hypothyroidism may be particularly subtle in the elderly. These symptoms of unsteady gait, weakness, and constipation are common in the elderly for a variety of reasons, but one of these reasons may be hypothyroidism. All of these symptoms should be investigated with a simple blood test to determine if an underactive thyroid is the reason for these troubles.

High Cholesterol

Sam is a forty-two-year-old accountant who is concerned about his overall health. He recently went for a routine checkup with his family doctor.

> *My cholesterol is very high. My doctor has told me to eat a low-fat diet, but I just keep on gaining weight and my cholesterol is still high. Could I have thyroid disease?*

Yes. An underactive thyroid may cause both a high cholesterol level as well as weight gain despite dieting. Getting treatment for hypothyroidism significantly decrease your body's cholesterol level, which in turn helps to prevent heart disease.

Other symptoms as a result of hypothyroidism range from voice changes, such as hoarseness, to a slow heart rate. You may experience muscle swelling or cramps (mainly in the arms and legs) or tingling in the fingers.

Once hypothyroidism is diagnosed, you may realize that you have many of these classic symptoms. These common symptoms—such as fatigue—are often overlooked because they are not specific to thyroid disease. Don't ignore what your body is telling you. If you are experiencing these symptoms you should be tested for thyroid disease with a simple blood test. Even if you don't have thyroid disease, your practitioner should take these complaints seriously and look for the root of these symptoms.

Causes of Hypothyroidism

Hypothyroidism may result from a variety of diseases of the thyroid. One of the most important causes is hereditary. If people in your family have a history of thyroid disease, you may be at risk too.

The second major risk factor for hypothyroidism is a problem with the production of thyroid hormone. As we discussed in the first chapter there are many different steps in the production of thyroid hormone, its release into the bloodstream as well as its proper conversion to its active form. Problems with any of these steps, as a result of a genetic defect, may lead to the underproduction of thyroid hormone.

Finally, an autoimmune inflammation of the thyroid may also cause slow destruction of the thyroid gland with the result of an underproduction of thyroid hormone. An autoimmune disease is a condition where the body does not recognize a part of itself as being familiar. For example, in autoimmune thyroid disease, the body's immune system tries to destroy the thyroid because it no longer recognizes it as a friendly part of the body. Rather, the thyroid is seen erroneously as a foreign intruder and the body attacks and slowly destroys it.

Other autoimmune diseases, such as prematurely graying hair (before the age of thirty), vitiligo (a skin disease that causes patches of white spots to form), systemic lupus erythematosus (also called SLE or lupus for short), diabetes, or rheumatoid arthritis are all diseases that increase the risk of thyroid disease up to 25 percent.

Thyroiditis

There are five different kinds of thyroiditis. Remember that *-itis* means inflammation. Thyroiditis is inflammation of the thyroid gland that may be associated with an underactive thyroid gland or hypothyroidism. Although each different type of thyroiditis may cause different symptoms, many times they can be quite similar.

In the case of thyroiditis, hypothyroidism is caused by destruction of the thyroid gland by an inflammatory process. When thyroid cells are attacked by the inflammation, these cells die. Without thyroid cells, the thyroid is no longer able to produce enough thyroid hormone to maintain the body's normal metabolism. Hypothyroidism or an underactive thyroid gland results.

Hashimoto's Thyroiditis

The most common cause of thyroiditis is called Hashimoto's thyroiditis. This form of thyroid disease may also be referred to as chronic lymphocytic thyroiditis. As we have already discussed, this autoimmune form of thyroiditis may run in families. Additionally, families that suffer from nonthyroid autoimmune disease, such as diabetes or rheumatoid arthritis, may also be at risk for the development of Hashimoto's thyroiditis.

Most people with Hashimoto's thyroiditis don't even realize they have any thyroid disease because the symptoms usually start out in a very mild form. Most often the thyroid grows slightly bigger, so that the thyroid appears bulky and larger. This enlargement of the thyroid gland is due to the inflammatory cells that destroy thyroid cells, resulting in long-term scarring.

When thyroid hormone can no longer be produced, hypothyroidism results. Again the symptoms are usually mild— fatigue, difficulty concentrating, and weight gain. But they can progress and be quite severe, affecting every organ system in the body, as described above.

Occasionally, if you have Hashimoto's thyroiditis, you may develop an overactive thyroid (hyperthyroidism), rather than the usual hypothyroidism that we just described. Too much thyroid hormone is the result of thyroid hormone release into the bloodstream as thyroid cells are destroyed. This hyperthyroid period is generally short, followed by a period of time when the thyroid functions properly. Sometimes, however, this period of normal thyroid function is short-lived. As scarring sets in, hypothyroidism results.

The diagnosis of Hashimoto's thyroiditis is simple—it's diagnosed by two blood tests. First, the routine thyroid function tests (in order to confirm that you have an underactive thyroid gland) and second, the thyroid antibody tests (in order to pin-point Hashimoto's thyroiditis as the cause of the hypothy-roidism) usually antimicrosomal antibody, but sometimes with antithyroglobulin antibodies. Antimicrosomal and antithy-roglobulin antibodies are highly specialized markers of thyroid autoimmune disease. Your body is producing antibodies (attackers) aimed at specific portions of the thyroid cells. The antimicrosomal antibody test is much more sensitive than the antithyroglobulin, therefore some doctors use only the former. These thyroid autoantibodies blood tests are high in about 95 percent of patients with Hashimoto's thyroiditis.

Although Hashimoto's thyroiditis is simple to diagnose, it can only be discovered if it is considered as a cause of your symptoms. If your doctor doesn't think of thyroid disease, then he doesn't test for it, which is tragic since it is such an easy disease to treat.

I have Hashimoto's thyroiditis and I also have a lump in my thyroid gland. Are the two processes related?

Although the thyroid gland enlarges with Hashimoto's thy-roiditis and sometimes even has exaggerated contours called bossilations, Hashimoto's thyroiditis does not form discrete nod-ules or lumps in the thyroid.

If you have Hashimoto's thyroiditis and a thyroid lump, it must be investigated fully to ensure that this nodule does not represent a cancer. This investigation is usually done by needle biopsy to prove whether or not the thyroid lump is benign or malignant. Although you are unlikely to develop thyroid cancer and Hashimoto's thyroiditis together, you are at increased risk for a special type of thyroid cancer called a lymphoma, which can be treated and cured if discovered early. Therefore, no thy-roid nodule should be ignored.

Painful Thyroiditis

The second type of thyroiditis is called subacute granulomatous thyroiditis, also sometimes called painful thyroiditis. Unlike most forms of thyroid disease, which are more common in women, this type of thyroiditis is seen in both men and women in equal numbers.

This disease usually starts out as a harmless viral illness, such as the flu or a cold, but ends up inflaming the thyroid gland and causing a thyroiditis. This type of inflammation is quite painful and you may find that the front of your throat is sore to the touch. Often this pain radiates to the jaw or ear. It can be confused with a whole host of other diseases including temporomandibular joint problems (commonly referred to as TMJ), ear infections, or even Strep throat. Sometimes only one lobe of the thyroid is affected causing pain and swelling on just one side of the neck instead of both.

In the situation where only one side of the thyroid gland is enlarged, the diagnosis of thyroid cancer may be mistakenly made unless your doctor is careful to obtain a thorough history, including recent viral illness. The diagnosis of painful thyroiditis is made by routine thyroid function blood tests, which may initially show an overactive thyroid. This overactivity is a result of the sudden release of a surplus of thyroid hormone into the bloodstream, as the thyroid is attacked by the virus. A radioactive iodine scan will show almost no concentration of the radioiodine by the thyroid cells because these cells are temporarily injured during the inflammatory process (see Appendix I—Diagnostic Studies.

Gradually the thyroid recovers and stops spilling thyroid hormone into the bloodstream. The thyroid gland begins to shrink and becomes less tender. If this shrinking happens on one side of the thyroid, but not on the other, a doctor may think that you have thyroid cancer unless you mention the painful initial swelling.

Gradually all swelling and pain disappear. Sometimes medications like aspirin or ibuprofen can be taken to help decrease the amount of pain. The thyroid cells recover and are usually able to produce normal amounts of thyroid hormone. Occasionally, however, the thyroid has been so destroyed that it never regains its ability to produce normal quantities of thyroid hormone. In this instance, permanent hypothyroidism results and replacement doses of thyroid hormone medication must be taken for the rest of your life. There is no way to tell who will eventually end up with an underactive thyroid gland. That's why it's so important to have routine visits with your doctor, to make sure that your thyroid gland is still functioning normally. This information is obtained by routine thyroid function blood tests.

Painless Thyroiditis

The third type of thyroiditis is called subacute lymphocytic thyroiditis, also sometimes referred to as painless thyroiditis. This type of thyroiditis may occur in women after they give birth. Painless thyroiditis is covered in more detail later on in chapter 8, "Pregnancy and Thyroid."

Reidel's Thyroiditis

The fourth type of thyroiditis is called Reidel's invasive fibrous thyroiditis. This is a very rare form of thyroiditis in which the inflammation of the thyroid gland causes it to merge with surrounding structures such as muscle and trachea. Actually, many people think that this disease is not a form of thyroiditis at all, but rather a rare type of low-grade tumor that happens to involve the fascia (or envelope) of tissue that surrounds the thyroid gland.

The thyroid gland itself becomes quite hard, like a rock, and it may be very difficult to tell if this rock-hard thyroid is a result of inflammation or cancer. Blood tests for thyroid function are usually normal except in the extreme cases where the inflammation has invaded the thyroid to the point where it can no longer function properly. In this situation, you may become hypothyroid.

A biopsy is necessary in order to distinguish this benign disease from cancer. However, since the thyroid gland in this illness is so hard, a fine needle aspiration biopsy may not be possible. Instead, the biopsy may have to be done in the operating room.

In the most severe forms of this disease, the thyroid gland becomes so tight and so hard that it may squeeze the trachea or breathing tube. In this instance, an operation may be necessary to remove the middle portion of the thyroid and remove this constricting ring. A complete removal of the thyroid gland cannot be performed because the thyroid blends with normal muscles and other tissues, making more extensive surgery quite dangerous. Once this little middle portion of the thyroid is removed, the windpipe is no longer being pressed on and you will experience an improvement in your breathing problems.

Acute Suppurative Thyroiditis

The last form of thyroiditis or acute suppurative thyroiditis is quite rare in modern times. It is caused by a bacterial infection in the thyroid that causes pus to collect and form an abscess within the thyroid gland. The bacterial infection may come from anywhere in the body and be carried in the bloodstream, or it may come from the throat itself. Because antibiotics are routinely used nowadays, we rarely see bacterial infections that progress and travel to the thyroid gland. In the few instances where it still occurs, antibiotics and surgery to drain the pus can provide a complete cure.

Other Common Causes of Hypothyroidism

Whenever the thyroid gland is removed completely by surgery because of a thyroid disorder, hypothyroidism results. If you have only half of your thyroid removed (and the other half that is not removed is normal), you can still produce enough thyroid hormone from the remaining half of the thyroid in order to function normally.

As we age, hypothyroidism becomes increasingly common, with 10 percent of all women over the age of fifty showing signs of a failing thyroid. Therefore, if you are older or if your remaining thyroid lobe is diseased in some way (Hashimoto's thyroiditis, for example) that remaining lobe of the thyroid may not provide enough thyroid hormone, thus resulting in hypothyroidism. If you've had half of your thyroid removed, you need to have regular checkups with your doctor for thyroid function blood tests in order to make sure that the remaining portion of the thyroid is functioning well. If it is not, you will need to start thyroid hormone medication.

Another common cause of hypothyroidism is the use of radioactive iodine. Some thyroid diseases such as Graves' disease (a form of hyperthyroidism) are treated with radioactive iodine. The radioactive iodine destroys the overactive thyroid cells, thus eliminating the source of the excess thyroid hormone or hyperthyroidism. This destruction sometimes results in hypothyroidism.

This type of hypothyroidism may be difficult to detect immediately, because there may be just a small amount of thyroid tissue that is not destroyed right away. This small piece of thyroid may produce enough thyroid hormone for the body for a little while. However, if this piece of thyroid burns out or gives up, hypothyroidism may result.

Because this hypothyroidism can occur anywhere from months to years after treatment with radioactive iodine, you may not immediately recognize the subtle symptoms of fatigue, weight gain, and difficulty concentrating. Therefore, if you have been treated with therapeutic doses of radioactive iodine, you should visit your doctor regularly and have routine thyroid function blood tests. By checking these blood tests once a year, hypothyroidism may be discovered in its earliest stages before you develop symptoms like fatigue and weight gain.

Finally, there are some rare causes of hypothyroidism related to brain diseases, also called secondary hypothyroidism. Disorders of the pituitary gland or hypothalamus portions of the brain may cause thyroid hormone deficiency in addition to other hormonal imbalances. This type of rare hypothyroidism can also be treated with thyroid hormone medication.

Treatment of Hypothyroidism

Although there are many different causes of hypothyroidism, the treatment is always the same. Once detected, hypothyroidism is extremely easy to cure with thyroid hormone medication.

Thyroid hormone medication is usually given in the form of

T4, also called levothyroxine. This drug is covered in detail in Appendix II, Thyroid Medications. It is safe, effective, and inexpensive if it is prescribed by a doctor who follows you closely and who is knowledgeable about the potential side effects.

Many people with hypothyroidism will need to take this medication for the rest of their lives. Thus, it is important to build a good relationship with your doctor and to be educated about the disease and its potential effects on your family.

Should Everyone with Hypothyroidism Be Treated?

If you have one or more symptoms of hypothyroidism as described above, treatment with thyroid hormone medication should be started. If you do not have symptoms, but hypothyroidism is discovered on routine blood tests, you should probably also be treated because you might become symptomatic in the future. Finally, if you have thyroid enlargement as a result of thyroiditis (but do not suffer from an underactive thyroid gland), you may also benefit from thyroid hormone medication in order to prevent further thyroid gland enlargement.

3

Hyperthyroidism

Hyperthyroidism (or an overactive thyroid) is relatively common in the United States. In fact, more than 2 million Americans suffer from this disease and the majority of these patients are women. Two percent of all American women will suffer from hyperthyroidism at some point during their lives.

The symptoms of an overactive thyroid may be subtle or full-blown—they can range from mild nervousness, weight loss, and insomnia to a dangerously fast heartbeat, which can be life-threatening. These symptoms are all caused by too much thyroid hormone in the bloodstream. There are many different reasons why there is too much thyroid hormone and, if recognized and properly diagnosed, all are curable.

Causes of Hyperthyroidism

There are many different causes of hyperthyroidism. The most common is Graves' disease, also called toxic diffuse goiter. We will discuss this disease in more detail later in this chapter.

Other causes of hyperthyroidism include toxic multinodular goiter (in which a person with a long-standing goiter develops several lumps within the thyroid that overfunction and produce too much thyroid hormone), a thyroid adenoma (a single lump within the thyroid gland takes control and overproduces thyroid hormone), and thyroiditis (inflammation of the thyroid gland that can result in an over-release of thyroid hormone into the bloodstream). Other rare causes include abuse of thyroid hormone medication (often from patients taking too many thyroid hormone pills because they mistakenly think it will help them lose weight; this is a fallacy—taking too much thyroid hormone can be dangerous and life-threatening), patients with metastatic thyroid cancer that overacts, or rare diseases of the ovaries or testicles that can cause the thyroid to be overstimulated.

Sarah is a fifty-five-year-old day-care worker who is physically fit and active. In addition to managing a group of preschoolers all day, she regularly swims at a local pool and walks two miles every morning before breakfast. One night while she was relaxing after work she began to experience alarming symptoms:

> My heart began to pound in my chest. I could feel each
> beat as if it were a drum. The beating became faster and
> faster until my head started to race and I became short of
> breath. I panicked and thought I was having a heart
> attack.

The body's heart rate is controlled by many factors, including thyroid hormone. If there is too little thyroid hormone, the heart beats slowly. If there is too much thyroid hormone, the heart beats too fast. In fact, the heart may not only beat faster, but the rhythm may become irregular. A rapid heart rate is called *tachycardia* and the most common abnormal rhythm is called *atrial fibrillation*. You may become acutely aware of your heartbeat and may even feel chest pain, shortness of breath, or faintness. Your blood pressure may also be elevated. President Bush's hyperthyroidism was diagnosed when his doctor noted that he had atrial fibrillation.

Jane is a twenty-five-year-old medical intern. She works long hours at the hospital and often has to stay up all night. She used to find this schedule quite grueling, but lately things have changed.

> *I feel great. I used to be so tired all the time. Now, I have extra energy. Those ten pounds that I've been working on for years have just faded without even dieting. I cleaned the whole house after work and tomorrow I'm going to clean out the garage!*

At first, you may feel terrific when you are hyperthyroid. The extra energy boost (especially if you've had a preceding period of hypothyroidism, or underactive thyroid) is a real plus. You are not bothered by the restlessness, rather you find it a positive.

Extra Energy Can Be a Problem

Amanda is a thirty-five-year-old mother of two who stays home to take care of her children. She is busy with car pool and after-school activities including everything from karate lessons to gymnastics. She has always been able to handle this busy pace with a calm attitude and good organizational skills. Recently, though, she feels like her schedule has become too much for her to handle.

*I feel restless all the time. I'm not sleeping at night and
I feel nervous and irritable. I've been fighting with my
husband and I have no patience for the kids. Something
is definitely the matter. I feel shaky and panicky, like I
can't control my emotions. It's like I have the world's
worse case of PMS! Even though I have all this nervous
energy, I can't concentrate and that makes me tired.*

Other Familiar Symptoms

Madeline, a thirty-six-year-old secretary, never had any weight
problems until recently. She had maintained the same weight
since high school. She gained about thirty pounds when she was
pregnant with her son, but was then able to lose this weight
later on with a regular program of diet and exercise.

*Lately I've been losing a lot of weight without even trying.
My appetite has actually increased and I'm eating more
than ever, but I still seem to be losing weight.*

The body's entire metabolism is increased with hyperthyroidism, therefore calories are burned faster. You may lose weight
despite eating excessive amounts of food. If you get used to this
increased caloric intake, you may continue eating large quantities
of food even after your hyperthyroidism is cured, putting you at
risk for weight gain and obesity.

Marilyn is a forty-year-old speech therapist in Florida who
works with emotionally disturbed children. She has always kept
an extra sweater in her locker at work just in case the air conditioner was too high, but she hasn't been using it. In fact, she has
the opposite problem.

*For the last three months, I've been perspiring a lot. Even
when the air conditioner is on, I'm still warm. I'm just
not comfortable anymore. I kick off all the covers and
keep the window wide open at night. My husband com-
plains I'm trying to freeze him to death! Maybe I'm going
through menopause but I'm only forty!*

The hot flashes associated with hyperthyroidism may be
similar to those experienced with hormonal changes, such as
menopause, but they tend to be more constant, rather than
coming on as brief flashes. This increased perspiration is due to
the increased heat of the body generated by a faster metabolism.

Many elderly patients do not have classic symptoms of
hyperthyroidism—such as nervousness and anxiety, but rather,
they experience subtle changes that they may not notice until
their hyperthyroidism is extreme.

Sandy is a sixty-year-old housewife with two grown children. She cares for her elderly mother, who lives in a nearby
senior citizens apartment house. Usually, Sandy stops by her
mother's apartment once a day—to help her with the laundry,
go grocery shopping, or to have lunch. One night she received a
frantic phone call from her mother, who had forgotten where
she had left her wallet. Sandy had to go over at 1 A.M. just to
calm her down and find her wallet.

*My mother is eighty years old and she's not what she used
to be. She has been losing so much weight and she doesn't
seem to have any appetite at all. She's up all night every
night since my father died and she just can't seem to get
any sleep. Lately she's been forgetful, and she left the stove
on by accident. I'm afraid she's going to harm herself. I*

feel so guilty about putting her in a nursing home, but I
just don't think she can manage on her own anymore.

Any elderly person with these symptoms of weight loss, insomnia, and forgetfulness should be thoroughly evaluated by a physician. Although there are many different causes of these symptoms—such as depression, cancer, and dementia—thyroid disease should also be considered as a potential diagnosis. A simple blood test for thyroid function will determine if the thyroid is the cause of these symptoms.

Hyperthyroidism may be particularly troubling in elderly who have a history of heart disease. With the extra workload demands put on the heart as a result of the increased body metabolism, the elderly are at risk for heart attack.

Effects on Eyes and Eyesight

Robin is a twenty-six-year-old paralegal who has worn contact lenses since she was sixteen. She rarely wears her glasses, except when she removes her contact lenses for cleaning. She began noticing her eyes were red and irritated; this persisted for two months. She tried cleaning her contacts more frequently and twice she even wore her glasses to work in order to give her eyes a break. But, nothing seemed to help.

My eyes are dry and red all the time. The lids are
swollen. Sometimes I can't even wear my contact lenses
because my eyes itch so badly.

Early eye symptoms, which occur in hyperthyroidism, are usually mild. If you develop only mild symptoms, you may be misdiagnosed with an eye allergy. You may find these symptoms to be particularly irritating at night, and environments with air conditioning or hot air heating as well as windy days tend to be particularly troublesome.

Occasionally you might develop double vision (*diplopia*), which is the result of scarring and swelling of the muscles that cause the eyes to move in their sockets. This scarring usually affects one side more than the other, rather than affecting both eyes in the exact same way. The enlargement of the tissue behind the eye can cause the eyeball to stick out and look very unnatural. This bulging eye (*exophthalmos*) causes disfigurement. The more the eyeball sticks out, the worse your symptoms become. In addition, the eyeball is very vulnerable to injury such as scratches or dryness, because it is not protected in the usual ways by the eye socket and eyelids. Swelling in the eye socket may actually contribute to loss of vision as pressure builds up on the nerve leading to the eye (the optic nerve).

You may notice excessive perspiration and your skin may feel warm to the touch. Your fingernails may become partially separated from your fingertips, a condition called *oncolysis*, or you may notice swollen fingertips (called *acropachy*).

Your gastrointestinal system may also be affected with diarrhea or an increased frequency of bowel movements. Your menstrual cycle may change with infrequent periods that are relatively light flow. In some severe cases of hyperthyroidism, you might experience weakness in the shoulders, hips, and thighs. Rarely, hyperthyroidism may be associated with *myasthenia gravis*, an autoimmune disease resulting in muscle weakness throughout the body. Men with hyperthyroidism may notice breast enlargement, called *gynecomastia*.

Untreated hyperthyroidism may lead to osteoporosis or thinning of the bones due to the body's increased metabolic demands on the bone. Even after treatment and cure of the hyperthyroidism, you can still be at risk for osteoporosis if the disease was undiagnosed for a long period of time. During this undiagnosed period, the bones were robbed of the calcium needed to grow strong. Exercise and a diet rich in calcium can help to prevent these long-term consequences.

Your thyroid itself may change with hyperthyroidism. It may grow large or it may develop a single lump or several lumps. These lumps may grow larger, while the rest of the thyroid gland shrinks.

Diagnosing Hyperthyroidism

In trying to make the diagnosis of hyperthyroidism, a doctor should ask you questions about your medical history and perform a careful physical examination with particular attention to weight, blood pressure, pulse rate and rhythm, thyroid gland, reflexes, eyes, skin, and lymph nodes.

The diagnosis of hyperthyroidism is made by thyroid function blood tests. In order to determine the exact cause of the hyperthyroidism, however, a nuclear scan is necessary (see Appendix I). If the thyroid gland is active on this scan then the most likely diagnosis is Graves' disease. Here, because the thyroid is overactive, the radioiodine is taken up by the thyroid gland and shows up positive on the scan.

If the thyroid is inactive on the scan, then the diagnosis is most likely thyroiditis (the thyroid cells are destroyed by the inflammation and thus do not appear to be active on scan).

Finally, one or more lumps may light up and show overactivity consistent with either a *toxic nodule* or a *toxic multinodular goiter*.

What Is Graves' disease?

Graves' disease is an autoimmune disease in which the body produces a false signal to stimulate the thyroid to produce too much thyroid hormone. This false signal is called an *antibody*. This disease may be caused by heredity and may run in families. In addition to the hyperthyroid symptoms noted above, you may notice thick or swollen skin over your shin bone (*pretibial myxedema*) as well as changes in your eyes, as discussed above.

About 20 percent of people with Graves' disease have only the eye symptoms and none of the other symptoms of hyperthyroidism. These patients have what is called euthyroid Graves' disease and do not require treatment for an overactive thyroid because they do not have the associated problems like weight loss, nervousness, and insomnia. Rather, they need specific treatment for their eye problems (see below).

How Is Graves' disease treated?

Once the diagnosis of Graves' disease is made, there are three treatment options: medication, radioactive iodine ablation, or surgery. Each option has pros and cons.

Medications

The most common medications used to control Graves' disease include methimazole and propylthiouracil (PTU). These medications are covered in detail in Appendix II. They do not control the hyperthyroidism immediately and up to six weeks may be required to stop overproduction of the thyroid hormone.

These medications are not without risks. There are a very small number of patients who suffer a severe reaction to the medication called *agranulocytosis*, where the body stops producing white blood cells that normally fight off infection. Without these cells, you are at risk for life-threatening infection called *sepsis*. If agranulocytosis is recognized early and treated, it is usually curable. With special medication to rebuild the body's immune system and white count, the majority of people make a full recovery.

The second major drawback of the medications used to treat Graves' disease is the fact that once the medication is stopped, over half of the people experience a relapse of hyperthyroidism, which requires restarting the medication.

Finally, because it is extremely important to take the correct dosage of the medication on a very strict time schedule (sometimes medication must be taken every six hours around the clock), many patients are not able to follow this rigid regimen and either take the medication incorrectly or not at all.

Despite these drawbacks, medication is still the recommended first step in controlling the hyperthyroidism of Graves' disease and the vast majority of people who are placed on these drugs experience an improvement in their symptoms.

If you are pregnant, think you might be pregnant, or are breast feeding a child, your doctor needs to know so that he can prescribe the correct medication at the proper dose. The severity of Graves' disease changes during pregnancy and you probably will need less of the antithyroid drugs as your pregnancy progresses. After delivery, however, there is usually an acute flare-up of the disease with worsening hyperthyroidism, requiring more medication to control it.

Radioiodine

The second treatment option in Graves' disease is radioactive iodine. The principle here is that enough radioactive iodine is given to a patient to destroy the thyroid gland and therefore prevent overfunctioning.

A single dose (between 3 and 12 mCi) of radioactive iodine is given orally in order to treat hyperthyroidism. Because it is impossible to give just enough radioactive iodine to destroy the exact right amount of thyroid gland—enough to cure the hyperthyroidism, but not enough to cause hypothyroidism—the result is usually an underactive thyroid.

This hypothyroidism may not occur for years because there may be a small amount of overfunctioning thyroid tissue after treatment. Eventually this overactive remnant will burn out and you will be left with a deficiency of thyroid hormone.

How long does radioiodine take to work?

Radioactive iodine takes several months to achieve its full effect, although symptoms should definitely improve after about four weeks. Additional antithyroid medications and beta blockers may be necessary to control the hyperthyroidism during this initial time period (see Appendix II).

How effective is radioiodine in curing Graves' disease?

Radioactive iodine is about 90 percent effective in providing a cure for hyperthyroidism. For the remaining 10 percent, a second dose of radioactive iodine is needed. Only a few percent of people fail this second dose and require surgery to remove the overactive thyroid gland.

Are there any risks associated with radioiodine?

Despite its efficacy, radioiodine has a bad reputation because people are fearful of undergoing this treatment once they hear the word *radioactive*. Their fears generally center around three topics. First, they are concerned that radioactive iodine may cause thyroid cancer. Second, they worry that radioactive iodine may cause other types of cancers, such as leukemia and lymphoma. Third, since most patients with Graves' disease are young women, these patients worry that the radioactive iodine will cause a problem with their ability to have children—either with infertility or in congenital malformations once they do become pregnant.

All three worries are unfounded. Thyroid practitioners today as well as the Food and Drug Administration agree that radioactive iodine constitutes a safe and effective treatment for hyperthyroidism. Multicenter trials looking at thousands of patients who have been treated with radioactive iodine have not found an increased incidence of thyroid cancer or any other type of cancer in patients who have been treated with radioactive iodine. Children and young adults who have undergone this form of treatment have also been carefully studied, and there do not appear to be any increased cancer risks.

Although radioactive iodine should never be given to a pregnant woman for fear of destroying the developing fetus's thyroid, radioactive iodine itself does not cause infertility or birth defects. It is currently recommended that you wait at least six months after undergoing radioiodine therapy before becoming pregnant so that all of the radioactive iodine is completely eliminated from the body, thus eliminating the risk to the fetus. Radioactive iodine should never be given to a woman who is already pregnant. And, if you are breast feeding, your breast milk will be contaminated by the radioiodine. If you want to continue to breast feed, you will have to pump milk and then discard it until your doctor feels it is safe for the baby to resume drinking the milk. How long you will have to do this depends on what dose of radioiodine you have received.

Are there any side effects of radioiodine treatment for hyperthyroidism?

Most of the radioiodine is concentrated in the thyroid itself, but some of it is picked up by the salivary glands around the jaws and under the tongue. Therefore, you may experience painful swelling and enlargement of these glands, which is treated by drinking plenty of fluids, sucking on lemon drops (in order to stimulate the flow of saliva), and occasionally pain medicine like aspirin.

Since the radioiodine is taken by mouth, you may experience nausea and vomiting soon after treatment. This side effect usually only lasts for a day or two.

Because it may take a few weeks after the treatment dose of radioactive iodine before there is a decrease in the blood level of thyroid hormone, you are at risk for a worsening of hyperthyroidism during this period. In many people, this increased period of hyperthyroidism may not be a problem; however, for patients with heart disease, this period of overactive thyroid hormone may put them at risk for a heart attack. The excess thyroid hormone may overstimulate the heart. For this reason, many practitioners prescribe antithyroid drugs for their patients who are about to undergo radioactive iodine treatment in order to prevent this "thyroid storm."

After undergoing radioiodine treatment for Graves' disease, you will need to follow the guidelines and precautions described in Appendix I, Diagnostic Studies, in order to avoid potential radiation exposure to close family members and friends. These precautions should be followed for one week if you receive between 3 and 6 mCi of radioiodine, two weeks for 6–12 mCi, and for one month if more than 12 mCi were administered.

Surgery

The third treatment option for Graves' disease is thyroid surgery. The principle here is that by removing the thyroid gland either completely or almost completely, the overproduction of thyroid hormone will be eliminated.

This surgical option is reserved for patients who cannot undergo treatment with either medication or radioiodine. If you are unable to take antithyroid medication because of an allergy or reaction to the medication (see above) or if the medication doesn't work well or if very large doses of medication are needed to control your hyperthyroidism, you may be a candidate for radioactive iodine or surgery.

Pregnant patients should not take radioactive iodine, as we have already discussed. Therefore, if you cannot take either medicine or radioiodine, you are a candidate for surgery. (Even pregnant women can safely undergo surgery.)

In the past, thyroid surgery for Graves' disease involved removing almost the entire thyroid, leaving only a small portion, to provide enough thyroid hormone for normal bodily functioning. The problem with this approach is that if too much thyroid is left in place, you may still suffer from hyperthyroidism and require additional treatment for cure. If too little thyroid remnant is left, you may develop hypothyroidism, necessitating taking thyroid hormone medication for the rest of your life.

Additionally, surgeons were reluctant to remove the entire thyroid because they wanted to minimize the complications associated with thyroid surgery, including damage to the nerves affecting the voice box or damage to the parathyroid glands, which control the body's level of calcium. Both potential complications are discussed in chapter 6. The risk of these complications is usually slightly higher during thyroid surgery for Graves' disease because the gland is often quite enlarged and contains an increased number of blood vessels, making the operation technically more difficult.

What causes the eye disease associated with Graves' disease?

If you have Graves' disease, your body may produce antibodies that attack the eye and cause eye changes such as protruding eyeballs, dryness, and the appearance of staring. The eye changes associated with Graves' *orbitopathy* can be very frustrating. The eye symptoms usually occur at the same time as the thyroid disease, however they may precede or follow the thyroid disease. Most people with thyroid abnormalities will never be affected by eye disease, and others only mildly so.

Although the incidence of eye disease associated with thyroid disease is higher and more severe in smokers, there is no other way to predict which thyroid patients will be affected.

Do the different treatment options for Graves' disease—medication, radioiodine, or surgery—affect Graves' eye disease?

While eye disease may be brought on by thyroid disease, successful treatment of the thyroid gland does not guarantee that the eye disease will improve as well. Although researchers are carefully studying potential reasons why one patient may have worse eye disease than another, we still don't know who is most susceptible. No particular thyroid treatment can guarantee eye improvements.

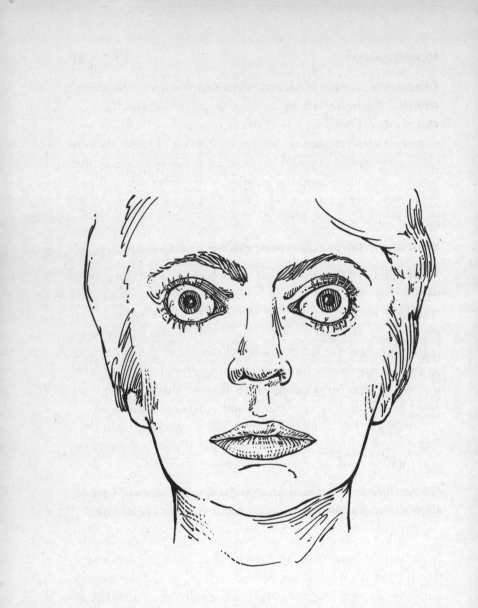

Woman's Face with Exophthalmos (bulging eyes) from Hyperthyroidism

*I have Graves' eye disease although I have been successfully
treated for Graves' disease of the thyroid. When will these
eye changes go away?*

Once inflamed, the eye disease may remain for several
months to as long as three years. Subsequently, there may be a
gradual or, in some cases, a complete improvement. While rare,
recurrence of the eye disease may occur if the thyroid becomes
underactive or overactive again. Thus, it is important to have
life-long monitoring after treatment for Graves' disease.

What can I do to improve the symptoms of Graves' eye disease?

Your condition should be monitored by an ophthalmologist
familiar with the disease and available treatments. Mild symptoms can often be successfully treated with lubricating eyedrops
and eye covers at night. Humidification of room air can prevent
drying of the eyes, and wraparound polarizing sunglasses can
also help to relieve glare.

Double vision or *diplopia* can be improved with special eye-
glass lenses called prism lenses. Temporary plastic prisms are available that are applied to glasses and changed as needed. Often this
double vision spontaneously improves. If there is no improvement
after several months, corrective eye surgery may be required.

Prednisone, a steroid medication, may be taken as a pill to
provide temporary relief from pain, swelling, and redness,
although side effects of the medication, such as weight gain,
may limit the use of this type of drug.

I have Graves' eye disease. Will I lose my sight?

Vision loss due to pressure on the optic nerve (the nerve
that controls eyesight) is the most severe form of the disease.

Fortunately this condition is very rare, affecting less than 5 percent of patients with Graves' orbitopathy. Treatment is with prednisone, radiotherapy, and/or surgery in order to restore vision. Overall, it is important to keep in mind that eye disease associated with Graves' disease will only improve gradually.

My eyes stick out a lot from Graves' disease. Nothing seems to help. Are there any other options for treatment?

If the eye condition does not improve or deteriorates despite treatment, surgery may be required. Pulled back and puffy eyelids can change your appearance and increase the risk of dryness to the lens of the eye or cornea. Corrective eyelid surgery can improve the problem through adjustable loosening of the eyelid muscles, as well as removal of scar tissue, excessive fatty tissue, and skin to place the eyelids in a more normal position. Surgery may also be necessary to correct diplopia when this problem has not resolved either spontaneously (within a few months) or with prism lenses. This surgery entails detaching and repositioning the eye-movement muscles on the eyeball to improve the way the eyes are lined up.

The enlargement of the tissue behind the eye may sometimes cause the eye to be pushed forward in the socket (*exophthalmos*). This condition can cause a serious cosmetic problem as well as endangering the eyeball, which is no longer protected in its socket. Swelling in the eye socket may actually contribute to vision loss as pressure increases on the optic nerve.

Surgical procedures relieve pressure on the optic nerve, improve vision, and allow the eye to settle back to a more normal position. This type of surgery, called *orbital decompression*, is useful if your eyeball protrudes so far forward that it is at risk for permanent vision loss. Sometimes careful resection of fat behind the eyeball is performed in addition to, or instead of, removing a portion of the eye socket bone. For most people, surgery is performed under general anesthesia and usually requires an overnight hospital stay.

Other Causes of Hyperthyroidism

What is the treatment for toxic multinodular goiter?

Toxic multinodular goiter is a condition where two or more lumps within the thyroid produce too much thyroid hormone. The result is hyperthyroidism.

The treatment for toxic multinodular goiter is usually radioiodine (see above). Occasionally, surgery will be required to treat toxic multinodular goiter if one of the thyroid lumps is suspicious for cancer.

What is the treatment for a toxic nodule?

A toxic nodule is a single thyroid lump that becomes over-active and produces an excess of thyroid hormone.

The treatment of a toxic nodule is surgery to remove the thyroid lobe that contains the nodule.

What is the treatment for thyroiditis?

There is usually no treatment for patients with thyroiditis who have hyperthyroidism, because most of the time, this type of hyperthyroidism gets better on its own within a few weeks to months. Most doctors do not prescribe antithyroid medications unless the hyperthyroidism is severe or prolonged. See also chapter 8, which discusses thyroiditis in women who have recently delivered babies.

4
Thyroid Nodules

A thyroid nodule is a lump in the thyroid. It is quite common to have a thyroid nodule. In fact, 3 to 5 percent of the world's population has thyroid nodules, the majority of which are benign. Most people with thyroid nodules don't even know they have them because these nodules do not cause any symptoms like neck pain or fever, but remain unnoticed until a physician finds them during a routine physical exam.

We do not know exactly what causes these nodules to form. Sometimes, a lack of iodine in the diet (see chapter 9) can cause thyroid enlargement. Other times, you may have a family history of benign thyroid nodules, thus making you more likely to develop a thyroid nodule also. You may already have a thyroid disease such as Hashimoto's thyroiditis, which can cause nodules to form. But, just because nodules can develop with this type of condition, doesn't mean that a nodule can be ignored. Each time a nodule is discovered it must be investigated as detailed below, and not just assumed to be a part of your previous thyroid disease history.

Carrie is a twenty-five-year-old woman who went to her gynecologist for a routine exam. During her visit, Carrie's doctor felt her neck while asking her to swallow a small sip of water. He found a lump on the right side of her thyroid that Carrie didn't even know she had.

A thyroid nodule can be felt by an experienced physician during a careful physical examination. Make sure to ask your practitioner (your internist, family practice doctor, or gynecologist) to check your neck at your next visit. Some thyroid lumps can even be seen just by looking at the front of your throat. Since the thyroid gland moves with every swallow that you take, a thyroid nodule will also move. This is the reason why some doctors may ask you to swallow while they are examining your thyroid gland. Some may even ask you to drink a glass of water during your neck examination in order to better check your thyroid.

Most thyroid nodules are not cancer. If you are younger than twenty or older than seventy you have a higher incidence of cancerous nodules than does the average person. In addition, there are more thyroid cancers in men who have thyroid nodules than in women.

Biopsies

Once a thyroid nodule is discovered, it should be biopsied in order to determine if it is benign or cancerous. The quickest and easiest way to perform a biopsy is called a fine needle aspiration biopsy. This technique uses a tiny needle (much smaller than the needle used to draw blood from your arm) placed into the thyroid nodule in order to draw out a few thyroid cells.

These cells are then examined under a microscope (just like a Pap smear examines cells from the cervix under a microscope) in order to determine if the nodule is cancerous. This test is generally done without any anesthesia since the needle is so tiny (remember, the technicians don't give you numbing medicine when they draw blood from your arm). Occasionally, if you are very fearful about the needle biopsy, a numbing medicine similar to the novocaine used at the dentist's office may be used. But the numbing medicine burns when it is injected into the skin just like a bee sting, so biopsies are generally performed without it. The results of this test are usually available within a few days.

If you have more than one thyroid nodule, this technique can be used on each of them whenever practical, with special attention to nodules that have recently grown in size. Then a cytopathologist (a physician who is trained to look at cell smears under the microscope) examines each slide and divides the diagnoses into four categories: 1) benign, 2) malignant, 3) indeterminate, and 4) nondiagnostic. We will discuss each of these categories in detail.

Benign

If the cytopathologist determines that a nodule is benign—and about three-quarters of all thyroid nodules will receive this diagnosis of goiter, also called nontoxic nodular goiter (NTNG for short)—we recommend a follow-up physical examination in six months. If the nodule is the same size or smaller at that time, we recommend yearly follow-up. If the nodule is larger in six months, a second biopsy is recommended and a course of action is determined depending on the results of this second biopsy: benign, malignant, indeterminate, or nondiagnostic.

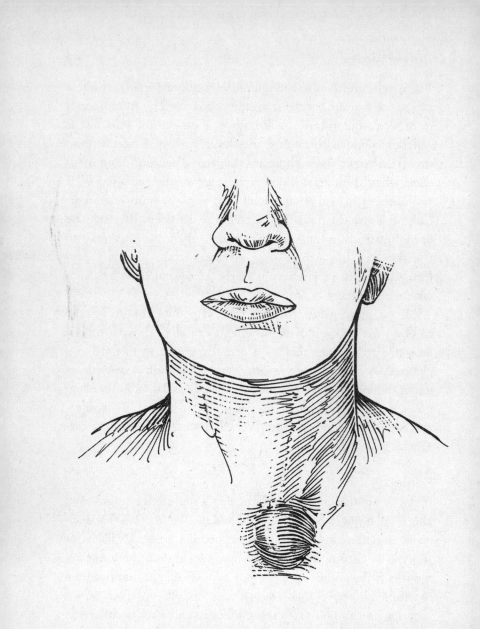

Lump in Woman's Throat

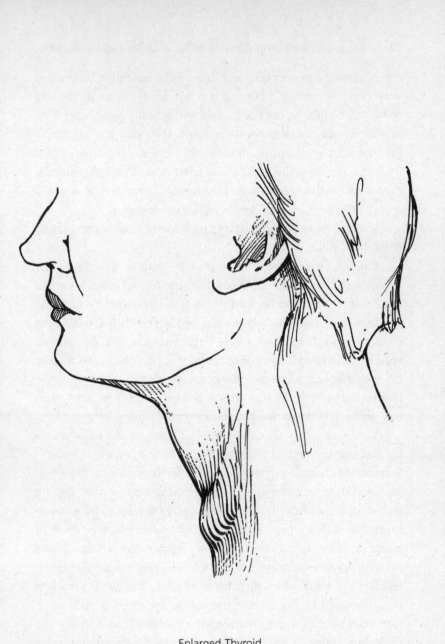

Enlarged Thyroid

No test is a perfect test, and fine needle aspiration biopsy can very rarely be wrong. About 1 percent of the time, the biopsy result will be benign, but the nodule will actually be a cancer. This mistake is called a false-negative result. How can the biopsy say that the lump is benign when it's really a cancer? It usually results from the fact that the needle was not inserted directly into the cancer. Either the needle missed the nodule or the needle sampled areas of the nodule that were benign, not cancerous.

If a nodule is very small, it is possible to miss it completely with the needle.

On the other hand, the larger a nodule is, the higher the probability of a sampling error. It's just like putting a needle blindly into a bruised apple. If it's a small crabapple with a big bruise, you're more likely to hit the bruise than if you put a needle into a big MacIntosh apple with a tiny bruise. An experienced practitioner can minimize the risk of missing the nodule or not sampling all areas. However, these risks can never be eliminated entirely. That is why it is so important to have a follow-up even if the initial biopsy report is benign.

There are a few situations in which we would recommend thyroid surgery even though we know that a nodule is benign. Sometimes a nodule can grow so large that it presses on the windpipe and/or the esophagus (the swallowing tube connecting the mouth to the stomach), causing difficulty breathing and or swallowing food. Your thyroid nodule may make you feel short of breath at night when you lie down because the weight of it is pressing on your windpipe. The thyroid nodule may also make you feel like solid food is difficult to swallow and like it's stuck in your throat when the thyroid presses on the esophagus. In these situations, thyroid surgery removes the pressure in this area of the neck. In addition, if these symptoms are ignored for many years (as the thyroid nodule grows slowly with time) you may have more severe difficulty breathing or swallowing, which might require emergency, rather than elective, thyroid surgery.

For example if your windpipe (trachea) is narrowed as a result of thyroid gland enlargement and you get a routine cold or flu, the mucous and phlegm caused by the cold may be just enough to close of the airway entirely, which would be an emergency situation.

Other people with benign thyroid disease may choose to undergo thyroid surgery because they do not like the way the thyroid gland looks. The thyroid may form a large lump in the front of your throat. Although you might not have any symptoms from the nodule, you may be self-conscious about the way the neck lump looks. Many people wear scarves or turtlenecks to try to hide their lump. Although thyroid surgery leaves a small scar, you may be happier with this scar than having a noticeable lump on your neck.

Malignant
If the cytopathologist determines that a nodule is a cancer, we recommend thyroid surgery to remove it (see chapters 5 and 6). The accuracy of a cancer diagnosis by needle biopsy is close to 100 percent.

Indeterminate
Next comes the indeterminate or suspicious category. This diagnosis falls somewhere in between benign and cancer. Some of these lumps are benign, others are precancers (meaning, if left untreated, they will develop into cancers), and others are cancers.

What should you do if your nodule falls into this category? Anywhere from 10 to 60 percent of these nodules are in fact cancers, but we still don't have a perfect way to tell which ones are benign short of performing thyroid surgery to remove the nodule completely.

One test used to try to improve the preoperative diagnosis is called a coarse needle biopsy. This is similar to the fine needle aspiration biopsy, but uses a much larger needle (see Appendix I). Because the needle is large, small nodules cannot be biopsied in this way. Also, if a nodule is very low in the neck or if a patient is obese, it may be difficult to perform this biopsy from a technical standpoint.

Since the needle is large, there is a risk of bleeding or injury to the windpipe or nerves controlling the vocal cords. However, these risks are quite small, less than 1 percent.

A coarse needle biopsy allows the physician to determine if your nodule is benign rather than premalignant (also called an adenoma) or malignant. It still cannot tell the difference between premalignant and malignant. If you look at all the patients who undergo thyroid surgery for a nodule that was diagnosed as indeterminate (suspicious) by fine needle aspiration biopsy, about 25 percent of them will actually have thyroid cancer. If both fine needle aspiration biopsy and coarse needle biopsy are used together to get a diagnosis, the cancer incidence rises to 40 percent. Although this number is an improvement over the results gained by using fine needle aspiration biopsy alone, it is still not perfect. Thus, some thyroid operations are still performed just to make a diagnosis of whether a thyroid nodule is benign or malignant. For practitioners who deal with thyroid disease on a daily basis, these numbers are frustrating, because we would like to operate only on people we know have thyroid cancer and avoid operations for benign thyroid disease.

Nondiagnostic

The last category of fine needle aspiration biopsy is called non-diagnostic. This is the result when there are not enough thyroid cells to make a definite diagnosis and occurs about 10 percent of the time. Occasionally, such a result may be due to a physician's inexperience with the biopsy technique; however, sometimes thyroid nodules can be filled with blood, hard material called calcium, or fluid and therefore only a sparse sampling of cells is obtained at biopsy.

Because up to 10 percent of these nondiagnostic thyroid nodules are cancers, we recommend a repeat fine needle aspiration biopsy in order to make a diagnosis, sometimes with a different size needle than was used for the initial biopsy (see coarse needle biopsy technique above). About half the time, we will be able to make a diagnosis of benign, suspicious, or cancer with this second biopsy. If a diagnosis still can't be made after the second biopsy, we generally recommend either very close follow-up (in three months) to see if the nodule has grown or thyroid surgery to make the definitive diagnosis.

Many times patients ask us if there are any medications that they can take to shrink their thyroid nodule and avoid thyroid surgery. Occasionally, if a fine needle aspiration biopsy is nondiagnostic, we recommend thyroid hormone medication in order to shrink the nodule (see Appendix I). This treatment is controversial because about one-third to one-half of all thyroid nodules shrink spontaneously without medication. Research reports are conflicted regarding whether or not thyroid hormone medication will shrink all thyroid nodules, although certainly, most practitioners agree that a certain subset of these nodules will shrink. The problem is we don't have a way to tell which nodules will respond to the medication and which won't.

Taking thyroid hormone medication is not without risks. We know that if you take doses of thyroid hormone that are too high, you can develop osteoporosis and/or heart disease. Therefore it is important to be carefully monitored on this medication (see Appendix II). If you are taking a dose that is right for you, there are no long-term complications with this medication.

If you are prescribed thyroid hormone medication, it may take several months to adjust the dose to your correct individual level. Therefore, we generally ask that you return for follow-up physical examinations at three and six months to determine whether or not your thyroid nodule has changed. If the nodule has grown larger, thyroid surgery is recommended to remove it in order to exclude a thyroid cancer. If the nodule has disappeared completely, the thyroid hormone medication is slowly tapered off and the thyroid gland is examined at three- to six-month intervals to make certain that the nodule does not reappear (requiring restarting the medication). If the nodule is the same size or slightly smaller, the medication may be continued for months or years (see Appendix II which covers the long term use of thyroid hormone medication).

It is important to note that although we understand that thyroid hormone medication shrinks some thyroid nodules, we do not know exactly its effect on the rest of the gland. We believe that taking thyroid hormone medication can probably prevent new nodules from forming.

Other Techniques for Diagnosis

Besides using the needle biopsy techniques described above, there are a few other tests that may be performed to evaluate the thyroid (see Appendix II). One of these tests is thyroid ultrasound. An ultrasound, or sonogram, is a test that looks at the thyroid without radiation. This test is very safe; in fact, it is the same type of test used on pregnant woman to look at the baby.

If you use ultrasound to examine people's thyroid glands, many small nodules can be identified that are too small to feel. It is estimated that by age fifty, 50 percent of people examined with a thyroid ultrasound will have nodules that are too small to feel. We are discovering more and more of these tiny nodules incidentally, when we perform neck ultrasounds for other purposes, such as an ultrasound to look at the carotid arteries to determine if a patient is at risk for having a stroke.

What is the significance of these nodules? Probably the vast majority of them are harmless incidental findings. If a nodule is too small to be felt (usually less than 1.5 cm, or three-quarters of an inch) and if you do not have any risk factors for thyroid cancer (such as a family history of thyroid cancer or exposure to radiation treatment—used to treat certain types of cancers such as Hodgkin's disease), we generally perform a follow-up physical examination in six months' time. If the nodule still cannot be felt at that time, we repeat the physical examination on a yearly basis. Other physicians advocate performing a biopsy on all of these tiny nodules. This is a controversial area and doctors are still exploring which treatment options are best.

If the nodule is greater than 1.5 cm, but still cannot be felt on physical examination, we recommend an ultrasound guided fine needle aspiration biopsy. This is the same as performing a fine needle aspiration biopsy (see above); however, using the ultrasound machine, a picture of both the nodule and the needle are obtained simultaneously. In this way, the practitioner can guide the needle into the nodule to be certain that the cells sampled are from the nodule itself and not from the normal surrounding thyroid tissue. The results of this biopsy will help determine if the nodule is benign or malignant.

In addition to ultrasound, some physicians rely heavily on a test called nuclear scanning (see Appendix I). This test is performed by giving an intravenous injection of a special radioactive substance, usually linked to iodine, which is rapidly taken up by the thyroid gland. Although this test uses radioactive material, it is very safe because only a very small amount of radioactivity is used and it is rapidly eliminated from the body. Because this radioactive substance is taken up by the thyroid, it can then be made into an image using a special camera. By examining the amount of radioactive substance that is taken up by a nodule (and comparing this amount to the amount taken up by the surrounding normal thyroid gland), we can determine if the nodule is functioning differently from this surrounding normal tissue. If a lot of radioactive substance is concentrated in the thyroid nodule, it is called overactive (hot). If only a little material is taken up by the nodule, it is called underactive (cold). If a nodule is hot, it is highly unlikely that it is cancer. On the other hand, if a nodule is cold, it may be a cancer. Although it is true that the majority of cancer nodules are cold, the majority of cold nodules, 85 to 95 percent, are benign. Therefore, we do not feel that this test is helpful in determining whether or not a thyroid nodule is cancerous.

All patients with a thyroid nodule should undergo thyroid function blood tests to determine if they have an underactive or overactive thyroid problem. Most patients with thyroid cancer do not have either hypo- or hyperthyroidism, rather they have normal thyroid function despite their cancer. If an underactive or overactive thyroid problem is detected, it should be treated (see chapters 2 and 3).

5
Thyroid Cancer

Thyroid cancer is relatively rare. There are about fourteen thousand new patients with thyroid cancer discovered every year and more than one thousand people died as a result of their thyroid cancer last year. Fortunately the vast majority of thyroid cancers are easily detected and highly treatable with an operation. There are four major types of thyroid cancer 1) papillary, 2) follicular, 3) medullary, and 4) anaplastic. The first two types, papillary and follicular, are sometimes grouped together and are referred to as differentiated thyroid cancer (each will be discussed in detail below).

In most instances, we don't understand why thyroid cancer develops in a particular person, but we do know of two main risk factors: first, exposure to head and neck radiation treatment and second, genetics, meaning that some types of thyroid cancer can run in families.

Type	Symptoms	Diagnosis	Treatment
Papillary	• Usually no symptoms • May have change in voice (hoarseness) or enlarged lymph glands	Fine needle biopsy	Surgery
Follicular	(same as above)	• Fine needle biopsy • May require coarse needle biopsy	Surgery
Medullary	• Usually no symptoms • In later stages may experience: - hoarseness - difficulty swallowing - difficulty breathing - enlarged lymph glands	• Fine needle biopsy • Calcitonin blood test	Surgery
Anaplastic	• Difficulty breathing • Voice change • Enlarged thyroid gland	• Coarse needle biopsy • May require biopsy performed in the operating room	• Early stage: Surgery • Late stage: Inoperable

Radiation

In the first half of this century, radiation therapy was used on children for a whole host of benign diseases, such as acne; scalp ringworm; enlarged tonsils; enlarged thymus or lymph nodes in the neck as a result of tuberculosis, whooping cough; and keloid scars. At the time, it was not known that the long-term effects of this radiation therapy to the head and neck area would cause thyroid cancers (called papillary cancer). If you received this type of radiation treatment, make sure to tell your doctor, who will want to examine your thyroid on a yearly basis.

We also know that people who were exposed to radiation as a result of nuclear weapons or nuclear plant accidents, such as the survivors of Hiroshima, Nagasaki, and Chernobyl are also at risk for the development of thyroid cancer. Because these cancers can develop decades after the initial radiation exposure, these survivors must also be followed closely.

If you have been exposed to these types of radiation, the thyroid is also at risk to develop benign thyroid lumps in addition to thyroid cancer. It is often difficult to distinguish between a benign area of the thyroid and a cancerous one because both conditions manifest themselves as thyroid lumps. When a cancer does develop in people who were exposed to radiation, it may be a more advanced form of the disease than a person without radiation exposure because of the difficulty in distinguishing between the benign and malignant nodules. Despite this difficulty, thyroid cancer patients who have been exposed to radiation are cured just as often as patients who were not exposed to radiation.

Family History

The other main risk factor for the development of thyroid cancer is a family history of thyroid cancer. For example, 5 percent of patients who develop papillary thyroid cancer have a relative who also had papillary thyroid cancer. With medullary cancer, this percentage can be much higher, as we will discuss below, and family members of patients with medullary thyroid cancer should be tested (with a simple blood test) to see if they are susceptible to the development of the disease.

Papillary Thyroid Cancer

Papillary thyroid cancer is the most common type of thyroid cancer, comprising about 70 percent of all thyroid cancers. It also has the best prognosis—most people with papillary thyroid cancer can be completely cured with surgery. After the operation, most people are cancer-free and go on to lead completely normal lives. Papillary thyroid cancer is more common than you might think. In fact, in many autopsy series (that is, if you examined all patients who died at a particular hospital because of any cause other than thyroid cancer) approximately 6 to 35 percent of these autopsies would reveal a papillary thyroid cancer. In other words, papillary thyroid cancer is frequently discovered in people who died of other causes. There are more than ten thousand new people with papillary thyroid cancer diagnosed in the United States every year. Most people develop papillary thyroid cancer before age forty, and it is much more common in women than in men, though we don't really understand why this disease affects predominantly young women.

The majority of people with papillary thyroid cancers do not even know they have the disease until a doctor notices a painless thyroid lump. Occasionally, a thyroid lump may be too small to feel, but instead, you or your doctor may notice an enlarged lymph node or gland in your neck that does not shrink. Remember that there are lymph nodes all over your body that help to fight infection. The ones in the neck can become enlarged ("swollen glands") when you have a sore throat. When your throat infection is better, the glands will shrink. If the glands do not become smaller in a few weeks, that could be a signal that the lymph glands are abnormal.

Most papillary thyroid cancers can be diagnosed by performing a fine needle aspiration biopsy—inserting a tiny needle into the thyroid lump or enlarged lymph node and drawing out a few cells. This technique is described in detail in appendix I. These cells are then examined underneath a microscope in order to identify characteristic features of papillary thyroid cancer cells.

The features that are unique to papillary thyroid cancer cells are changes within the nucleus or main warehouse of the cell. Normally this nucleus is dark and round, but with papillary thyroid cancer there can be large clear areas within the nuclei that look like "Little Orphan Annie" eyes. These changes are called "optically clear nuclei" and are, for the most part, diagnostic of papillary thyroid cancer.

In addition, some nuclei may appear to have a line or groove in them. This appearance is called "nuclear grooving" and is also highly diagnostic for papillary thyroid cancer. Other features of the fine needle aspirate which would suggest papillary thyroid cancer but which are not diagnostic for it include: the presence of psammoma bodies (spiral rings of calcifications) or the presence of papillary fronds, which look like the fronds of a fern plant.

This type of biopsy is over 90 percent accurate if the above-mentioned features are present and if the biopsy is performed by an experienced practitioner and examined under the microscope by a skilled doctor.

There are no medicines that you can take to cure papillary thyroid cancer, so surgery is really the only treatment option.

Most people can be cured by an operation to remove the thyroid gland. Once the diagnosis of papillary thyroid cancer has been made by fine needle aspiration biopsy, surgery is indicated in order to remove the tumor.

Currently, there is still a lot of debate about how much surgery should be performed for papillary thyroid cancer. Remember that the thyroid gland is shaped like a butterfly. Removing one wing or lobe of the gland is called a lobectomy. Removing almost the entire gland on both sides is called a subtotal thyroidectomy, and removing the entire gland on both sides is called a total thyroidectomy.

The extent of the surgery performed really depends on individual features of the tumor as well as judgment intraoperatively by your surgeon in order to determine if the papillary thyroid cancer has spread to the opposite lobe or to the lymph nodes in the neck. More extensive surgery is associated with higher complication rates (see chapter 6) and thus many surgeons who are inexperienced in thyroid surgery choose to perform lesser operations in order to decrease the complication rates. In general, our preference is to remove the entire thyroid gland in order to prevent the cancer from returning or spreading to the opposite side. Sometimes we are asked to see patients who have had a lobectomy as a second opinion. Three options are available to these patients: 1) no further treatments; 2) reoperation to destroy the remaining thyroid lobe or; 3)radioiodide treatment to destroy the remaining thyroid lobe. If your thyroid cancer was small and not aggressive (see below) we generally don't advise more treatment. If the cancer was advanced, however, then we advise option two or three.

If you have had a history of head and neck irradiation, removal of the entire thyroid gland is especially important because you may have lumps on both sides of your thyroid gland (see above). Cancer may occur anywhere within the thyroid, not just in the large lumps.

There are many different classifications for scoring and grading papillary thyroid cancer. This "staging" system is needed in order to determine your prognosis and to help define what type of surgery you need. One of the most commonly used staging systems is called TNM, which stands for Tumor size, presence or absence of lymph node metastases (meaning has the cancer spread to the lymph Nodes in the neck), and presence or absence of distant Metastases (meaning has the cancer spread beyond the neck to other areas of the body like the lung or bone). Based on these three categories, you can be assigned a Stage of 1, 2 ,3 or 4. Stage 1 is the best category and the best prognosis, and Stage 4 is the most advanced category. This staging system was introduced in 1987 by the International Union Against Cancer and adopted by the American Joint Commission on Cancer.

Another popular staging system is AMES (Age, Metastases to different sites other than neck lymph nodes, Extent of primary tumor, and Size larger than 5 cm—about 2 inches).

We prefer the AGES (Age, Grade, Extent, and Size) scoring system, first developed at the Mayo Clinic in the 1980s because it is useful in predicting outcome as well as the extent of surgery that should be performed. AGES is a complicated scale that requires a health-care practitioner who is expert in thyroid disease in order to be accurate, but when used properly, is extremely accurate in predicting survival from papillary thyroid cancer.

If a patient is forty years of age or older, his age is multiplied by 0.05 in order to give the A score. Grade refers to how closely the tumor resembles normal thyroid tissue. If the tumor is similar to normal thyroid tissue, it is considered to be well differentiated and no points are assigned. Depending how different the tumor is from normal tissue, a score of 1, 2, or 3 may be assigned. Next is the extent of the tumor. If the operating surgeon feels that the tumor is invading adjacent structures outside of the thyroid gland such as muscle, the windpipe (trachea) or swallowing tube leading to the stomach (esophagus), a score of 1 is given. If the patient has known metastatic disease at the time of the operation, such as thyroid cancer that has traveled to the lung or bones, they receive a score of 3. Lastly, the largest size of the tumor in centimeters is multiplied by 0.2 for the size score. All of these points are added together to form the total AGES score.

The majority of people with papillary thyroid cancer will have an AGES score of less than 4. In these instances, the chance that you will die from papillary thyroid cancer is almost zero. But if the score is 4 or greater, there is a 50 to 75 percent chance that you may die from thyroid cancer over the ensuing fifteen years. This score is extremely accurate and was devised from studying thousands of patients with papillary thyroid cancer.

In addition, as long as the surgeon has successfully resected all of the papillary thyroid cancer in patients with an AGES score less than 4, it does not make a difference in terms of survival how much thyroid tissue was removed at operation. In other words, as long as the cancer is completely removed (remember that up to 70 percent of the time the cancer can be in both lobes of the thyroid gland), it makes no difference in survival whether a portion of the thyroid or the entire thyroid is removed.

It is interesting to note that the presence or absence of

lymph node metastases is not included in the AGES scoring system for papillary thyroid cancer. In other words, in terms of survival, thyroid cancer that spreads to the lymph nodes of the neck does not impact on survival at all. This is a difficult concept for many people to understand. Most people think that positive lymph nodes give you a worse prognosis. This is certainly true for many common types of cancer such as breast, colon, and lung cancers, but is not true for papillary thyroid cancers.

If neck lymph nodes are enlarged as a result of papillary thyroid cancer, you will need to have them removed in an operation called a modified radical neck dissection. This operation involves removing the lymph nodes along one side of the neck. After the operation, this area of the neck is usually numb because the nerves to the skin in this area are purposely severed in order to remove the diseased lymph nodes. Other than this numbness, there are no long-term effects of having these lymph nodes removed.

Sometimes both the left and right sides of the neck must be cleared of lymph nodes. If this is the case, two separate operations are performed about two months apart. This delay is to allow time for healing on one side before beginning the operation on the opposite side. Performing the lymph node dissection on both sides at the same time could lead to unnecessary swelling (edema) of the head and face. Edema can occur if sufficient time is not allowed between operations for alternate pathways of blood flow to form in order to drain the head and neck area.

There is still a lot of controversy about the way you should be followed by your physician after papillary thyroid cancer surgery. There are many different tests available to try to identify cancer recurrences in the neck and elsewhere in the body such as lung or bone.

One of the best and still least expensive tests is a careful physical examination by a practitioner skilled in thyroid disease. Because papillary thyroid cancer tends to spread to lymph nodes in the neck rather than other far-away areas such as lung or bone, a careful physical examination can easily detect a recurrence in a neck lymph node(s). A small operation can remove these affected nodes and provide a complete cure.

Other tests used to detect metastatic disease include radioactive iodine scanning, ultrasound, serum thyroglobulin levels, sestamibi scanning, and thyroglobulin RT-PCR. Each one of these methods has some good points and some bad ones, and they are described in detail in appendix I.

Many people want to take an active role in their recovery from thyroid cancer. We advise a healthy lifestyle and diet. Exercise regularly. Decrease your alcohol consumption. Quit cigarette smoking. Eat a diet which is low in fat, high in fiber. These changes are recommended to reduce many types of cancers, not just thyroid. A positive attitude can help your overall health as well as your long-term outlook.

In addition to these suggestions, we know that if you have undergone surgery for papillary thyroid cancer, you will benefit from taking thyroid hormone medication after your operation, for the rest of your life. The thyroid hormone tricks the brain into thinking that enough thyroid hormone is being manufactured by the thyroid gland, therefore shutting down the brain's production of TSH (thyroid-stimulating hormone, which normally encourages the thyroid to manufacture thyroid hormone).

If TSH is left at high levels, it will stimulate both the remaining normal thyroid as well as the thyroid cancer and metastases to grow and enlarge. Taking thyroid hormone medication suppresses TSH and thyroid cancer growth is checked. In order to maintain a dose of thyroid hormone that is right for you, blood tests for thyroid function will need to be checked periodically. Generally, these blood tests are performed every two months in the beginning until a stable dose has been achieved and then every six months for two years and then yearly after that.

We used to believe that patients with a history of thyroid cancer needed to be maintained on very high doses of thyroid hormone medication. These high doses may have some undesirable and dangerous side effects, such as the development of heart disease and/or osteoporosis, as described in Appendix II. New studies, however, have shown that these high doses are not needed to prevent cancer recurrence in most instances. Rather a dose of medication close to the normal range may be just as effective in preventing recurrent or metastatic disease. Ask your doctor what is your correct individual dose.

If Your Thyroid Cancer Returns

If your doctor discovers a new lump in your neck or if one of your blood tests or X-rays are abnormal, the cancer may have returned. This happens very infrequently, but if it does, there are many treatment options available. If a cancer recurrence is detected in your neck lymph nodes, the best course of action is usually an operation to remove the affected node or nodes (see above).

Other treatment options include radioiodine therapy. This treatment is similar to a radioiodine scan (described in detail in Appendix I); however a much larger dose of the radioactive iodine is given. Radioactive iodine is given orally and this iodine is taken up by thyroid cancer metastases and the radioactivity destroys them (without harming other parts of your body).

One problem with this treatment is that normal thyroid tissue attracts the radioactive iodine much more efficiently than does thyroid cancer metastatic disease. Therefore you can only undergo this type of treatment if you have had your entire thyroid gland removed. If you've been treated with removal of just part of your thyroid gland, the remaining normal thyroid gland will interfere with this therapy. Thus, you must undergo an operation to remove the remaining gland or receive initial radioactive iodine treatment with a low dose of medication in order to wipe out the normal thyroid before proceeding with a larger dose to eradicate the thyroid cancer. If you have not had your entire thyroid removed, but need to be treated with radioactive iodine, you can receive this initial lower dose about six to eight weeks after your thyroid surgery.

If you are treated with large doses of radioiodine to destroy thyroid cancer metastases, you will need to be hospitalized and placed in isolation for several days after taking this medication in order to minimize the risk of radiation exposure to others. If other people are exposed to your radiation for a prolonged period of time, they could have damage to their thyroid glands.

The radioactive iodine is passed out of the body through the gut, bladder, mouth, and skin. Therefore all bodily eliminations, such as stool, urine, saliva, and sweat, are potential forms of contamination. If you are undergoing radioiodine treatments, you must be hospitalized in a special isolation room where all of your bodily secretions may be disposed of properly. You will be served your meals on paper plates with disposable utensils. Your urine and stool will be collected and disposed of in proper radioactive waste containers. Your bedsheets will be specially laundered. Personal items such as pillows, stuffed animals, or needlepoint should not be brought into the isolation room since these items will become contaminated with radioactivity. Newspapers, magazines, and paperback books are allowed because they can be thrown away.

All nurses, doctors, and housekeeping personnel who enter your hospital room must wear a special badge to monitor the amount of radiation that they are exposed to. Only brief visits are permitted.

After the hospital's radiation safety officers have determined that the level of radiation is low enough for discharge (using a portable machine that measures radioactivity), you will still have to closely follow the precautions outlined in appendix I for approximately one month.

Right now, it is unclear who should have their thyroid cancers treated with radioactive iodine. We know that the majority of patients with thyroid cancer have a very slow growing form of the disease that is not aggressive. These patients are completely cured by thyroid surgery alone. Only a minority of patients have the more aggressive form of the disease, which is potentially lethal.

Because radioactive iodine treatment has some major drawbacks—it is expensive, time consuming, and requires you to be isolated for several days after the treatment (see above). It also requires you to be off your thyroid hormone medication for at least one month prior to treatment (thus allowing symptoms of hypothyroidism—fatigue, weight gain, and exhaustion; particularly felt by the elderly—see also the section about preparation for radioiodine scanning), it is difficult to decide who should undergo this form of treatment.

We currently reserve radioiodine therapy for patients with

aggressive disease who we feel are increased risk for recurrence and metastasis.

In the future, a new type of medication called recombinant TSH may be widely available to use instead of making patients stop taking their thyroid hormone medication. Recent reports have indicated that this medication is only being used for diagnostic radioiodine scans, not for radioiodine therapy. Initial studies show that the recombinant TSH may not produce as accurate a scan as the traditional way to prepare for this test, which involves stopping your thyroid hormone medication (see Appendix I).

Follicular Thyroid Cancer

Like papillary thyroid cancer, follicular thyroid cancer is classified as differentiated thyroid cancer, which means that it arises from the thyroid cells in the thyroid. Follicular cancer in general accounts for about 25 percent of the thyroid cancers that are diagnosed and is usually a more aggressive form of cancer than the more common papillary thyroid cancer.

Follicular thyroid cancer is most often discovered as a painless lump in the thyroid. This type of cancer usually occurs after the age of forty and is much more common in women than in men.

Unlike papillary thyroid cancer, it can be difficult to diagnose without performing surgery. A fine needle aspiration biopsy often cannot distinguish among the precursor to follicular cancer (called a follicular adenoma), follicular cancer, and a completely benign condition called nontoxic nodular goiter.

Even a coarse needle biopsy cannot always provide an answer since it is only able to distinguish a follicular neoplasm (which includes both adenoma and cancer) versus nontoxic nodular goiter about 40 percent of the time. This difficulty in diagnosis is one of the most frustrating areas for physicians who study thyroid disease, because it means that often a thyroid operation is the only way of definitively deciding if a thyroid nodule is a cancer.

Follicular thyroid cancer can be completely cured by surgery. However, like papillary thyroid cancer, there is a lot of controversy about how much thyroid should be removed. Not only is the diagnosis of follicular thyroid cancer difficult to make before an operation, it can be difficult to make during the operation as well. The diagnosis of follicular thyroid cancer is usually only made after the operation, when the pathologist can thoroughly inspect and examine multiple portions of the thyroid nodule under the microscope. This elaborate inspection can sometimes take up to a week to perform. Unless we definitely know the diagnosis is a thyroid cancer during the operation, we will only remove one half (lobectomy) of the thyroid gland. Remember that removing both sides of the thyroid gland is associated with increased complications (see chapter 6), therefore we reserve this operation for cancer patients only when the benefits outweigh the risks. Thus, the most common operation performed for follicular thyroid cancer is a lobectomy or removal of one half of the thyroid gland.

Follow-up and treatment after you have undergone thyroid surgery for follicular carcinoma is similar to that detailed above under papillary thyroid cancer. Unlike papillary cancer however, which can metastasize to the lymph nodes in the neck, follicular cancer tends to spread to different sites, such as the lungs or bones.

If metastatic disease affects the bones, for example the spine, it weakens the bones and can cause a fracture. Depending on the location of the metastasis, this can have catastrophic effects. For example, if the vertebral column is involved, collapse of these bones could lead to paralysis. Treatment with radioactive iodine or external radiation therapy may be necessary to stabilize the bone and decrease pain from the cancer invasion.

The overall survival rate of patients with follicular thyroid cancer is about 75 percent after ten years. However, this figure can be as low as 40 or as high as 85 percent depending on individual features of the tumor, such as whether or not the tumor invades blood vessels (more aggressive) versus the capsule surrounding the cancer (less aggressive).

Medullary Thyroid Cancer

This type of thyroid cancer is completely different than the papillary and follicular types that we've been discussing. Medullary thyroid cancer does not arise from the thyroid cells themselves, but rather from the specialized "C-cells" that are in between the thyroid cells. These C-cells are also sometimes referred to as parafollicular cells. They are found mostly in the upper and middle parts of the thyroid.

C-cells produce a substance called calcitonin, which can serve as a blood test marker for medullary thyroid cancer. Although we know that calcitonin is somehow involved in the body's regulation of calcium, we do not know its exact function. We do know that people who have had their thyroids removed surgically do not require replacement of this calcitonin substance for normal function and healthy life.

There are four different types of medullary thyroid cancer:

1: Sporadic The first type is called sporadic. This name refers to the fact that there is no family history of medullary thyroid cancer and that the patient who develops this disease will not pass it on to their children.

2 and 3: MEN 2A and MEN 2B The second and third types are called MEN associated medullary thyroid cancer. MEN stands for Multiple Endocrine Neoplasia, which are a group of tumors affecting hormone glands that are passed on from one generation to the next. Although there are several different types of MENs, MEN 2A and MEN 2B are the ones associated with medullary thyroid cancer.

MEN 2A is a hereditary syndrome in which affected patients suffer from medullary thyroid cancer, tumors of the adrenal gland (the adrenal glands are specialized endocrine glands located on top of each kidney), and tumors of the parathyroid glands (four glands near the thyroid gland that control the level of calcium in the bloodstream).

MEN 2B patients usually have medullary thyroid cancer and tumors of the adrenal gland, but do not have problems with their parathyroid glands. Instead, these patients all have characteristic bumps on the end of their tongue, called mucosal neuromas. These bumps are also found on the underside of the eyelid and throughout the gut. Their faces are distinguished by thick lips and thickened eyelids.

4: Familial The fourth type of medullary thyroid cancer is called familial type, which means that the thyroid cancer is passed genetically through a family, but not in association with the other endocrine tumors that occur in the MEN syndromes.

Because there are so many different types of medullary thyroid cancers, they can occur in people of different ages. The MEN-associated type usually occurs in younger patients, while the non-MEN familial and the sporadic types occur usually in patients in their forties or fifties. Unlike differentiated thyroid cancer, which usually affects women, medullary thyroid cancer affects women and men equally.

Most patients with medullary thyroid cancer do not have any idea that they have the disease until their doctor notices a painless lump in their thyroid. A few people with more advanced forms of the disease can have hoarseness, difficulty swallowing (especially solid foods), and difficulty breathing. Others people have enlarged neck lymph nodes, indicating spread of the tumor to these nodes. Occasionally some patients will also have diarrhea, possibly due to the elevated calcitonin levels in the blood produced by the tumor.

The diagnosis of medullary thyroid cancer is usually suggested by abnormal cells obtained from a fine needle aspiration biopsy. These cells can then be specially stained for calcitonin in order to confirm the diagnosis. Blood tests showing an elevated calcitonin and CEA level also help in identifying this cancer.

Once the diagnosis is made, it is important to search for other associated tumors, such as adrenal and parathyroid. A careful family history should be obtained and special importance given to relatives who died from unknown causes at an early age, perhaps an aunt who died during childbirth or a brother who died while undergoing anesthesia for a routine operation. Often a rare adrenal tumor called pheochromocytoma can cause massive elevations in blood pressure and sudden death, especially with external stress such as childbirth or anesthesia. If an adrenal tumor is found, it will require operation prior to thyroid surgery in order to ensure safe blood pressure levels during the thyroid cancer operation.

Because this disease tends to involve both lobes of the thyroid gland with multiple tumors in the hereditary forms of the disease, the operation of choice is a total thyroidectomy plus lymph node dissection both in the center of the neck as well as the side(s). This operation is described above in the section on papillary thyroid cancer.

The best prognosis is associated with the familial form of the disease, the worst with the MEN 2B–associated form, while the MEN 2A and sporadic forms have prognoses somewhere in between. There is an 80 percent ten-year survival for the very earliest forms of disease that are confined to the thyroid gland without metastasis, but that figure drops to about 25 percent for patients with disease metastatic to lymph nodes or distant sites such as the lung, liver, and bone.

For people who undergo thyroid surgery for C-cell hyperplasia (which is the precursor to medullary thyroid cancer), the survival rate is 100 percent. An important issue in the discussion of medullary thyroid cancer is the question of whether future family members may develop this form of cancer. Remember that three out of the four types of medullary thyroid cancer are hereditary.

In the past, we have used a special test called a calcium/pentagastrin stimulation test in order to identify who had an early form of medullary thyroid cancer or the precursor to this type of cancer, called C-cell hyperplasia. This test involves the intravenous injection of two substances, calcium gluconate and pentagastrin, both agents that stimulate the C-cells of the thyroid to produce calcitonin. Serial blood tests to check for calcitonin levels are obtained prior to the test and at one, two, three, and five minutes after the injection. Family members with elevated calcitonin levels are considered to be at risk for medullary thyroid cancer and prophylactic thyroid surgery is recommended.

Currently, we have a better way to determine which family members are at risk for medullary thyroid cancer. A special genetic test called direct DNA testing is available. This is a blood test that identifies a defect in the genetic material that causes medullary cancer to form.

Although we have identified many defects or mutations that cause medullary thyroid cancer, we have not identified all of them. Therefore this test is only useful if you have a family member with medullary thyroid cancer who tests positively. Then your family can be screened for this mutation. Family members who test positively are candidates for prophylactic thyroid surgery. If a patient with known medullary thyroid cancer tests negatively for these mutations, then their family members must be screened the old-fashioned way with the calcium/pentagastrin test as described above.

If you have a family history of medullary thyroid cancer or other endocrine tumors, it is important to be screened for medullary thyroid cancer with a simple blood test. By discovering the disease in its earliest forms, total cure is possible.

After your operation, you will be followed by careful physical examination, as well as blood tests to determine your calcitonin and CEA levels. If these levels rise, some surgeons would advocate a repeat operation to clear out any new neck lymph nodes that have been invaded by cancer. The location of these lymph nodes (either right or left side) may be determined preoperatively be obtaining blood samples for possible elevated calcitonin levels from both the right and left sides of the neck through a small tube inserted in the groin (femoral) vein, which is threaded up to the neck area.

Occasionally, if you cannot undergo another operation because the tumor is has spread to many different organs in the body, additional therapy with radiation or chemotherapy is used to improve symptoms. However, these forms of nonoperative treatments are not curative, and the disease will eventually spread further, causing death.

Anaplastic Cancer

Anaplastic thyroid cancer, which is also called undifferentiated thyroid cancer, is relatively rare. Although, earlier in this century, this disease comprised up to one-fifth of all cases of thyroid cancer, that figure is now down to about 5 percent of all thyroid cancers. Even though anaplastic thyroid cancer is decreasing in frequency, we don't know the reason for change.

We do not know what causes anaplastic thyroid cancer, although some people believe that it develops from other less aggressive thyroid cancers that suddenly become out of control for unknown reasons.

Anaplastic thyroid cancer is more common in older people with an average age of about sixty. It is more common in women than in men.

The symptoms of anaplastic thyroid cancer are usually noticeable right away. Most patients initially complain of difficulty breathing—either shortness of breath or noisy breathing—as well as changes in their voice, usually hoarseness. These changes are the result of the rapidly growing cancer pressing on the windpipe and invading the nerves that enervate the voice. Additionally, most patients notice a large and rapidly growing lump in the front of their neck.

The diagnosis is made by a careful history and physical

examination as well as a biopsy—usually done with a large needle. The biopsy is essential in order to tell the difference between this type of thyroid cancer and other forms, such as medullary cancer or thyroid lymphoma. A blood test for calcitonin can also be performed in order to rule out medullary cancer as the cause of the thyroid enlargement.

After the diagnosis of anaplastic thyroid cancer has been established, it is important to see how extensive the disease is. A CT scan of the neck and chest can show how large the tumor is; whether or not it is invading the nearby muscles, trachea, and esophagus; as well as determine if the disease has spread to the lungs. A flexible laryngoscopy can determine if the vocal cords have been affected by the cancer (see appendix I).

In the very lucky situation where the cancer has been identified at its earliest stages, surgery can be attempted to remove the thyroid gland. However, the vast majority of patients have advanced disease that is inoperable. The five-year survival from this type of cancer is less than 10 percent, with most patients dying within just a few months of the diagnosis.

Treatment with radiation therapy or chemotherapy may shrink the tumor slightly and make breathing easier in those patients who are suffering from shortness of breath. Occasionally, a tracheostomy (a surgically cut hole in the patient's windpipe) may allow easier breathing, but will not cure this aggressive form of cancer. With advances in research, we hope that additional treatment options will be available soon.

6

Thyroid Surgery

If you need thyroid surgery, it is important to know what to expect. Write down a list of questions before you see the doctor so you will remember what to ask. If you have additional questions after meeting with your physician, call or set up a new appointment to meet with him or her in person. Following are some of the most frequently asked questions about thyroid surgery.

How long will I be hospitalized?

You will be admitted to the hospital on the morning of your surgery. Although an overnight bed is automatically reserved, you may choose to go home on the same day after a six-hour period of observation in the recovery room.

What type of anesthesia will I have?

The majority of centers in the United States offer only general anesthesia, however a few are now offering local anesthesia.

With general anesthesia, you are completely asleep during the operation. With local anesthesia, your neck area is numbed with a medication similar to the novocaine used at the dentist's office so that you are awake during the surgery. Mild sedatives may be given through your intravenous line in order to keep you comfortable and calm. If you choose to have local anesthesia, you will be in close communication with your surgeon throughout the operation. To choose the method of anesthesia that is right for you, discuss these options with your doctor.

Will I have a scar?

Yes. All surgery causes scarring, and how you form a scar depends on how your body heals. There are, however, some techniques that surgeons use to minimize scaring, such as a small incision size, careful incision placement, and hypoallergenic suture material to avoid an inflammation and infection. Many people ask if there are any creams they can use (such as aloe, vitamin E, or cocoa butter) that will improve the appearance of the scar. There are no known creams to minimize scarring, but these creams or other common body lotions may alleviate the itching sometimes associated with healing during the first few months after surgery.

You might notice bruising around your incision or upper chest and slight swelling above the scar when you are upright. In addition, the scar may become pink and hard. This hardening will peak at about three weeks and may result in some tightness or difficulty swallowing, which will disappear over the following two to three months. With most people, the scar fades and becomes difficult to notice by about six months after surgery.

Will I have pain after the operation?

All operations involve some pain and discomfort. Our goal as surgeons is to minimize this discomfort. At the time of operation, your doctor may inject long-acting numbing medication to the thyroid area in order to minimize postoperative pain. The effect from this medication usually lasts about eight hours.

Although you should be able to eat and drink normally after the operation, you may have some dull pain with swallowing.

We suggest that you take Torodol (a prescription medication similar to ibuprofen), ibuprofen, or acetaminophen every four to six hours for the first forty-eight hours after the surgery. It is important to take the medication before the pain is severe since the pills take approximately thirty to forty-five minutes to have an effect.

After surgery, you will tend to hold your head in one position because it can be uncomfortable to turn your neck normally. This position can cause a muscle imbalance that can lead to muscle tension and headache. The most effective way to prevent headache is to exercise your neck. Two exercises are particularly helpful. 1) Touch your chin to your chest and then raise your chin to the ceiling. 2) Roll your head in slow circles, first clockwise, then counterclockwise. These range of motion exercises will help stretch out your muscles and reduce cramping.

If your operation was done under general anesthesia, you may feel like you have phlegm in your throat. This is usually because there was a tube in your windpipe while you were asleep that caused irritation. You will notice that if you cough, very little phlegm will actually come up. This sensation should subside about four or five days after the surgery.

When will I know the findings of the surgery?

During the operation, your surgeon will sometimes consult with a pathologist who will provide a preliminary diagnosis. However, the final pathology report requires careful study of the thyroid tissue that was removed. Therefore, the final report is usually not available until about one week after the operation. Occasionally, the pathology report may take weeks to finalize if special studies need to be performed on the removed thyroid tissue.

Will I have stitches?

Yes. The majority of surgeons use dissolvable stitches that don't need to be removed. We, however, favor using a single nondissolvable suture that is removed immediately prior to leaving the hospital. We think that this method causes less reaction (absorbable sutures create an inflammatory reaction in the skin in order to dissolve) and thus less scarring. The result is a less noticeable scar.

We also use a protective strip of clear glue called colloidium to act as a bandage. With this type of dressing, you can shower and wash your hair as usual, as long as you are careful not to soak or scrub the incision. The collodium will turn white and start curling up at the edges after four or five days. When this happens, you can pull it off or wait until it falls off on its own. If you experience itching once the colloidium is off, you may apply body cream or hand lotion to the scar.

Will I have any physical restrictions after my surgery? When will I be able to go back to work?

Swimming is the only major restriction. In general, your activity level depends on the amount of discomfort you experience.

Many people play golf or tennis within a week after the operation. You will be able to return to work within the first two weeks. For safety reasons, driving is not recommended until you can comfortably turn your head.

You should feel overall improvement every day after surgery. If you have questions regarding your progress, call your surgeon. In fact, a phone call to your surgeon's office the first two days after your surgery to report how you feel can help your surgeon monitor your condition. You should schedule a routine follow-up appointment with your surgeon for about three weeks after surgery.

What complications can occur?

As with any surgery, there is always the risk of bleeding and infection. Bleeding after the surgery is generally quite rare, occurring in less than 1 percent of patients. The bleeding usually occurs within the first six hours after the operation, and if discovered in the recovery room, requires a repeat operation to stop the bleeding. Infection is also quite rare occurring in about 0.1 percent of patients undergoing thyroid surgery. A wound infection is treated by opening the incision, draining any accumulated pus, and starting antibiotics.

Two complications are unique to thyroid surgery and these include injury to the nerves affecting the voice or injury to the parathyroid glands (four small glands that sit near the thyroid gland and control the level of calcium in the bloodstream).

In less than 2 percent of thyroid operations, the nerves that control the voice are affected by the surgical removal of the thyroid gland. When this occurs the main difficulties are projection of the voice and difficulty producing high-pitched sounds. These changes are usually described as a "hoarse" voice. Generally your voice will be better in the mornings and "tire" toward the end of the day. This can last for variable periods of time, but generally not longer than three months. These changes are such that you or a close family member might notice the difference in your voice, but a stranger meeting you for the first time would not notice anything unusual. Voice changes are usually temporary, so your voice will return to normal within several weeks; permanent voice changes are rare.

The other complication that is specific to thyroid surgery is injury to the parathyroid glands during operation. These are four delicate glands that are located near the thyroid. Since the parathyroid glands control calcium levels in the bloodstream, injury to these glands results in as a lowered calcium level. This dysfunction is usually temporary and causes the blood calcium to drop below normal (called hypocalcemia).

Symptoms of hypocalcemia include numbness and tingling around your lips, hands, and the soles of your feet. You may experience a "crawling" sensation in your skin, muscle cramps, or severe headaches. These symptoms appear between one or two days after the surgery. It is rare for them to begin after three days.

Hypocalcemia is treated with calcium tablets (available over the counter, we prefer the brand-name Oscal), specifically two tablets of Oscal 500. It is a good idea to purchase Oscal tablets before your surgery so that you can take it at home. If you feel you need it, take the calcium (there is no danger in taking the tablets even if you do not need them) and at the same time call your surgeon to confirm the need. The symptoms of tingling/numbness should subside within twenty to thirty minutes of taking the tablets. Once you start taking the calcium, you should repeat the dose whenever the symptoms return. This may mean that you are taking as many as two tablets every three hours.

It is important that you keep you surgeon informed. The hypocalcemia should disappear in about seven to ten days. If it does not, tell your physician, who may prescribe vitamin D tablets in order to reduce your symptoms, if you do not respond to the calcium alone. If the parathyroids do not regain their normal function within thirty days, calcium and vitamin D tablets may need to be taken on a permanent basis.

Both of these complications (voice changes and parathyroid injury) occur in less than 2 percent of patients overall and are directly related to the operative experience of the surgeon. Although the risk of these complications cannot be eliminated entirely, it can certainly be minimized by an experienced thyroid surgeon.

7

Thyroid Disease in Infants and Children

Diseases of the thyroid gland that affect infants and children can be divided into three categories: 1) hypothyroidism (underactive thyroid), 2) hyperthyroidism (overactive thyroid), and 3) thyroid lumps or nodules with the potential for thyroid cancer. The first two illness, hypo- and hyperthyroidism have very different causes, symptoms, and treatments for the newborn baby versus the older child.

Hypothyroidism in the Newborn

"When my baby was born, the nurses took a drop of blood from his heel and sent it to the State Newborn Screening Program. The doctors told us it was to check for thyroid disease. How can a newborn baby have thyroid disease?"

Congenital hypothyroidism, or an underactive thyroid, in newborn babies is a significant health problem. If undetected, these children grow up to be severely intellectually delayed. They also suffer from stunted growth. This impairment in intellectual and physical development as well as some component of deaf-mutism is sometimes referred to a cretinism. The only way to prevent these problems is to detect congenital hypothyroidism early and to treat it.

Because we are able to screen for hypothyroidism by placing a drop of blood from a newborn baby's heel on a piece of filter paper, we have made significant advances in identifying these children and providing them with treatment at an early stage, before the illness is irreversible. A joint committee of the United States and Europe now routinely screens millions of newborns worldwide for thyroid and other metabolic abnormalities and identifies approximately two thousand hypothyroid infants per year.

The most common cause of hypothyroidism in a newborn baby is a thyroid gland that is in an abnormal location. Instead of being located in the front of the throat, which is its normal position, abnormal development during the fetal period causes the thyroid to end up in a different place, like at the back of the tongue. Thyroid tissue that is located in an abnormal position often does not produce normal amounts of thyroid hormone. The result is an underactive thyroid. Finally, a newborn may have hypothyroidism as a result of goiter or benign enlargement of the thyroid gland if the expecting mother takes antithyroid drugs to treat hyperthyroidism during pregnancy (see chapter 8). The abnormally large thyroid gland or goiter may not produce thyroid hormone efficiently, resulting in low levels of thyroid hormone in the bloodstream or an underactive thyroid.

After an incorrectly positioned thyroid gland, the next most common cause of congenital hypothyroidism is failure of the thyroid gland to form at all. This absence of thyroid tissue is called *agenesis*, meaning failure to form.

The treatment of hypothyroidism in the newborn is to give thyroid hormone medication. If the medication is given before the baby is three months old, the vast majority of these children will have normal IQs. Whereas if the condition is unrecognized and treatment is begun after three months of age, the majority of children will have IQ scores that are lower than normal.

Premature babies who are hypothyroid are at increased risk for cerebral palsy and intellectual retardation when compared with premature babies with normal thyroid function. Studies are currently being conducted to see if giving these hypothyroid babies small doses of thyroid hormone medication will improve their neurologic outcome.

Ectopic Thyroid

During pregnancy, the thyroid gland begins to develop during the tenth to twelfth weeks. This time period at the end of the first trimester is critical for the production of thyroid hormone. The thyroid gland begins as a group of cells in the back of the mouth area near the base of the tongue. As the fetus develops, this group of cells moves down the neck and forward to its eventual location in the front of the throat. This movement is important because it explains two developmental abnormalities that are sometimes seen in children called *ectopic thyroid* and *thyroglossal cysts*. Sometimes the thyroid never makes it to its final destination and a small leftover piece of it is found along its track, like at the back of the tongue (ectopic or lingual thyroid) or high up in the neck (thyroglossal cyst). This abnormally positioned thyroid gland may not function as well as a thyroid gland in its normal position, thus the newborn baby may be at risk for the development of hypothyroidism.

The most common location for ectopic thyroid tissue is the front of the throat. Sometimes when the thyroid is developing in the fetus and traveling to its proper location in the front of the throat, a little thin piece of thyroid tissue can be left behind and form an extra strip in the front of the throat just above the thyroid gland, called the pyramidal lobe. If you picture the thyroid as shaped like a butterfly with each wing representing a lobe of the thyroid, then the pyramidal lobe sticks up from the center of the thyroid like a large antenna. This pyramidal lobe is seen in about half of all people, and isn't a problem.

The second most common location for this ectopic thyroid tissue to be found is at the base of the tongue, way in the back of the throat (lingual thyroid). This type of ectopic thyroid tissue can cause problems if it is not treated because it can grow and create difficulty breathing and swallowing. Most of the time this problem is discovered in childhood, and is rarely found in adults.

In about 70 percent of people with thyroid tissue in the back of their throats, lingual thyroid, this little bit of thyroid tissue may be the only thyroid tissue they have. In other words, the thyroid gland never made it to the correct location in the neck and became stuck at the base of the tongue.

If your child has lingual thyroid tissue, he or she can become hypothyroid because this little bit of thyroid tissue cannot make enough thyroid hormone. Other times, there may be enough production of thyroid hormone initially, but, as your child grows, this amount may no longer be sufficient. These children are risk for the acquired development of hypothyroidism later in life.

It is important to determine if this lingual thyroid is your child's only thyroid tissue, because if this tissue is surgically removed your child may have no other source of thyroid hormone, thus becoming hypothyroid. A nuclear scan (see appendix I) will determine whether or not there is additional thyroid tissue in the proper location.

Because ectopic thyroid tissue represents normal thyroid tissue that is just in the wrong location, it may still potentially develop the same diseases that normal thyroid tissue can; namely it can develop into a cancer or enlarge to form a goiter. Any enlarged ectopic thyroid tissue needs to be examined not only by nuclear scanning (as above), but also by biopsy.

Surgery may be necessary to remove this ectopic thyroid tissue if it enlarges and interferes with speaking, breathing, or swallowing, or if it is suspicious for a cancer. If a cancer is discovered in this location (because it is causing these symptoms), it is treated in the same way that any other thyroid cancer is treated (see chapter 5). If the thyroid tissue is discovered by accident (at the dentist's office for a routine visit, for example) and is not enlarging or causing symptoms, your child may be placed on thyroid hormone medication in an attempt to shrink the tissue or prevent it from enlarging in the future.

Thyroglossal Duct Cysts

"I was bathing my toddler in the bathtub the other day and I noticed a bump in the front of her throat that I've never seen before. What is it?"

The second developmental abnormality that may occur in children is the thyroglossal cyst. As the thyroid develops in the fetus, it descends down a tunnel or "duct" from the base of the tongue to its normal position in the front of the throat. Normally, the leftover tunnel then disintegrates and there is no longer a connection between these two points. If this duct does not close, however, a persistent tract can remain that may appear as a small lump in the front of the neck.

The majority of these abnormalities are discovered in early childhood, in toddlers. Most babies tend to be chubby, especially around the head and neck areas. When babies lose this extra fat as they grow older, these thyroglossal cysts are usually first noted. They are found equally as often in boys as in girls. Often they become infected, turning red and swollen. Pus may drain spontaneously out of a tiny pore in the center of the lump.

It is important to distinguish between a thyroglossal cyst and a thyroid lump. Your doctor will ask your child to swallow some water and also to stick out his tongue. A thyroid lump or nodule will move when the child swallows, whereas a thyroglossal cyst will move when the child sticks out his or her tongue, since the thyroglossal cyst represents a persistent tract from the base of the tongue.

If a thyroglossal cyst is discovered as a result of infection, it will have to be cut open and drained. This incision will usually be performed in the office with a small amount of numbing medicine and takes about ten minutes. In addition, antibiotics may be necessary to clear the infection faster.

Only after the infection has resolved can the cyst be removed entirely with a small operation. Most children will require general anesthesia for this operation, which carefully dissects the path of the cyst up to its origin and removes this tract in its entirety. Because this tract contains small amounts of normal thyroid tissue there is a potential for this tissue to become cancerous. If a cancer is discovered, treatment and prognosis is the same as for other thyroid cancers (see chapter 5).

Hypothyroidism in Children

"My child is very short. He used to be in the ninetieth percentile for height, but now he's so short that he's off the curve. My husband and I are not tall people, but he's now the shortest one in his class by far. What's the matter?"

Although there are many causes of short stature, *acquired juvenile hypothyroidism* is one that needs to be considered in all children who fail to grow at a normal rate. Children who become hypothyroid after the age of three do not suffer from the severe mental retardation that infants with unrecognized hypothyroidism do. They do however suffer physical growth delays, particularly with regard to bone growth and development. In adolescents who are hypothyroid, the onset of puberty may be delayed.

The most important step in making the diagnosis of hypothyroidism is the discovery that a child is growing slowly. Each time your child visits the pediatrician, his height is recorded. These values are then placed on a graph to compare with a normal range for that particular child's age category. If a child who has previously been growing normally slowly begins to fall outside the normal range, then hypothyroidism should be suspected. Routine thyroid function blood tests will make the diagnosis of hypothyroidism.

The most common cause of acquired hypothyroidism is Hashimoto's thyroiditis. This disease may affect a little more than 1 percent of schoolchildren in this country. It is more common in boys than in girls and is usually associated with a family history of thyroid illnesses.

In addition to an underactive thyroid, your child may also have other underactive endocrine glands such as the pancreas, pituitary, or adrenal glands. This is particularly important if your child already has diabetes, and all children with diabetes should be screened for thyroid disease with a simple blood test.

Because the symptoms of this form of hypothyroidism are subtle and progress slowly, this diagnosis may be difficult. One of the most common causes of hypothyroidism in a child is an abnormally located thyroid gland (see the section on ectopic thyroid, above). This incorrectly located gland may make enough thyroid hormone for the child to develop for several years, but with increased growth and age, this thyroid tissue does not provide enough thyroid hormone for normal development. Other causes of acquired hypothyroidism include rare genetic conditions or prescription drugs that may have an antithyroid effect.

Once recognized through the use of routine thyroid function blood tests, the treatment for acquired hypothyroidism is simple, namely thyroid hormone medication. Although most children who are started on thyroid hormone medication catch up to their normal and expected height, children who have suffered from untreated hypothyroidism for many years may never reach their full height potential.

Hyperthyroidism in the Newborn

It is very unusual for a newborn baby to have an overactive thyroid. The most common cause however, is an infant who is born to a mother with Graves' disease. It doesn't matter if that mother had a history of Graves' disease that was successfully treated long before she became pregnant or if she had active Graves' disease during her pregnancy. These babies are at risk for hyperthyroidism. The mechanism is the transfer of the mother's thyroid stimulating antibodies via the bloodstream and through the placenta to the fetus where they stimulate the baby's thyroid (see chapter 8).

The symptoms of hyperthyroidism may begin even before your baby is born. A rapid fetal heart rate may be detected by your obstetrician at a routine prenatal visit. These babies are often born prematurely and weigh less than normal infants do. Most babies show the bulging and protruding eyes found in adult Graves' disease. Other babies may fail to thrive and are unable to gain weight despite adequate nutrition. Some of these hyperthyroid infants are colicky and cry all the time.

Once this disease is suspected, the diagnosis is confirmed by routine thyroid function blood tests and is easily treated by using antithyroid drugs such as propylthiouracil or methimazole (see Appendix II). The overall prognosis for these children is quite good and the majority can have their medication tapered after a six-month course. If the hyperthyroidism is severe and untreated, however, up to one-quarter of these infants may die due to complications of the disease.

Hyperthyroidism in Children

"My child is hyperactive. He wasn't always that way. He used to be a good student and a good kid, but recently things have changed. The teacher says he can't sit still in class. He never finishes his homework. Even when I help him, he can't seem to concentrate for more than a few minutes. The doctor said he may have attention deficit disorder. I just can't believe it. He used to be so normal."

Although there are many causes of hyperactivity in children, hyperthyroidism is one that can be easily diagnosed and treated. Therefore all of these children should be tested for thyroid disease in order to rule out this possibility.

After the age of five, Graves' disease is the most common form of hyperthyroidism. Although children experience the exact same symptoms as adults (see chapter 3), this illness is difficult to diagnose because many parents and medical practitioners do not think of it.

The nervousness and restlessness seen in the adult Graves' patient may be thought of as hyperactivity in a child with undiagnosed Graves' disease. Often these children are labeled with attention deficit disorder and are treated incorrectly. Their difficulty concentrating and insomnia may translate into poor school performance. Many parents believe that these children are lazy, not motivated, or perhaps are taking illicit drugs. Other children have uncontrolled emotions, moodiness, and temper tantrums and are referred to a child therapist for counseling. Many children with Graves' disease have an excessive appetite, although most do not gain weight normally because of their increased metabolism.

A careful history, physical examination, and routine thyroid function blood tests will confirm the diagnosis of hyperthyroidism. Unlike adult hyperthyroidism where there are many causes of this disorder, Graves' disease represents the vast majority of case of childhood hyperthyroidism. Therefore additional testing with nuclear scans is seldom required.

The treatment for Graves' disease in children is the same for adults with this illness. Treatment options include antithyroid medication, radioiodine treatment, and surgery (these options are discussed in detail in chapter 3).

Many parents are reluctant to use radioiodine treatment in children because they are fearful of the radioactivity. But the fears regarding radioactivity as a cause of childhood cancer are unfounded. Similarly, the children born to parents who had been treated in childhood with radioiodine do not have an increased incidence of congenital malformations including genetic abnormalities when compared with the general population. Studies have followed children treated with radioiodine for more than forty years and it appears to be a safe and effective form of treatment. Surgery is reserved for those children who are unable to take antithyroid drugs due to a reaction or for children whose parents refuse to give them radioioidine treatment or for the small percentage of children who are treated with radioiodine and develop a recurrence of hyperthyroidism.

Although hypothyroidism (which is easily treated with thyroid hormone medication) may develop in children who have had their thyroids destroyed by radioiodine or surgical removal, all children with Graves' disease are at risk for a relapse of hyperthyroidism. Thus, every child who has had Graves' disease needs to be followed for the rest of his life in order to detect recurrent or new thyroid abnormalities and treat them in a timely fashion.

Finally, these children must be followed closely in terms of diet and weight gain. Many of them are used to eating large portions of food like they did before the hyperthyroidism was diagnosed and treated. After therapy, their metabolism will return to normal. If they continue to consume large quantities of food, they will become obese. Proper nutritional counseling is essential in all of these children.

Thyroid Cancer in Children

As discussed in the introductory chapter as well as chapter 5, thyroid cancer is a relatively rare disease with only about fourteen thousand new cases discovered in the United States each year. In children, however, this type of cancer represents about 3 percent of all cancers seen in childhood and adolescents.

We know of two main risks factors for the development of thyroid cancer in children and these are a history of radiation exposure to the head and neck region and/or a family history of thyroid cancer. Because the thyroid gland grows rapidly in children, increasing its size more than ten times from infancy to adulthood, young people are especially susceptible to the damaging effects of radiation exposure. This radiation may be a result of a medical treatment for another form of cancer, such as leukemia, or it may be the result of exposure due to nuclear weapons or accidents.

In the first half of this century, radiation was used commonly to treat benign conditions like tonsillitis or acne. By the 1950s however, the relationship between radiation and thyroid cancer was recognized and this treatment was abandoned and reserved only for therapy of cancers. The period of time between the initial exposure the radiation and the subsequent development of thyroid cancer is variable, with an average of nearly nine years. Thus, any child exposed to radiation needs to be followed closely for suspicious thyroid nodules. This surveillance needs to be lifelong, as some of these children will develop thyroid cancer many decades after the radiation. Many doctors recommend that children exposed to radiation be treated prophylactically with thyroid hormone medication in an effort to prevent the subsequent development of thyroid cancer.

The second major risk factor for the development of thyroid cancer in children is a family history of thyroid cancer. This risk applies mainly to patients with a family history of medullary thyroid cancer, covered in chapter 5. However, a small proportion of papillary thyroid cancer, which is the most common form of thyroid cancer, may also run in families.

Thyroid cancer is more common in girls than in boys, and the average age for discovery of childhood thyroid cancer is sixteen years. Most children do not have any symptoms. Rather, their pediatrician discovers a thyroid lump on a routine physical exam. Since a thyroid lump in a child is more likely to be a cancer than a thyroid lump in an adult, all thyroid nodules discovered in children must be investigated thoroughly. Often children will not have a thyroid lump, but rather have enlarged lymph nodes in their neck (swollen glands) as a result of thyroid cancer that has spread to the lymph nodes. (More information on how to test the thyroid lump or lymph nodes to see if they contain thyroid cancer is presented in chapter 5.)

The treatment of these childhood cancers is an operation to remove the thyroid gland (see chapter 5). Because children often have more than one thyroid cancer within the thyroid gland, the entire gland should be removed. In addition, since many of these children also have a high incidence of metastases to the neck lymph nodes, a modified neck dissection should be performed on the side where the cancer was discovered. If enlarged, cancerous lymph nodes are discovered on both sides of the neck, then these lymph nodes should be removed in two separate operations.

Even though children who have thyroid cancer often have cancers that are more extensive than adult patients have, the fact that the cancer has spread to the neck lymph nodes does not generally mean a worse prognosis. In fact, children with thyroid cancer have a better prognosis than do adults with the disease.

Treatment after surgery with radioactive iodine is controversial, but is generally advised for children with aggressive forms of cancer. Almost one-quarter of children develop cancer recurrences in neck lymph nodes, thus aggressive follow-up is required to catch these recurrences early and treat them with either repeat surgery or radioactive iodine.

All of these children will need to be placed on thyroid hormone medication for the rest of their lives since their entire thyroid has been removed. There are also data to support that thyroid hormone medication in properly controlled dosages prevents cancer recurrence and spread, so the outlook for the majority of these children is excellent.

8

Thyroid Disease and Pregnancy

Since thyroid disease is common in women (remember that thyroid lumps may occur in up to 5 percent of women), many pregnant women also suffer from thyroid disease. Thyroid illness can play a major role in infertility, fetal abnormalities, stillbirth, and premature labor. Babies who are born to mothers with thyroid disease may have hypothyroidism or hyperthyroidism, which if unrecognized may have profound impact on their future intellectual, emotional, and physical development.

In addition, many instances of postpartum depression are actually due to thyroid illness in the postpartum period, which can be easily diagnosed and treated. Therefore it is critical that physicians be able to recognize, diagnose, and treat women with thyroid disease during pregnancy in order to minimize these complications. If you have or have had any thyroid problems, you should alert your obstetrician, because many of the tests and medications used for nonpregant woman may be unsafe to take during your pregnancy.

The thyroid gland enlarges in pregnant women. In ancient

Egypt, this thyroid growth was actually a crude pregnancy test. The Egyptians would tie a reed around a woman's throat and if, with time, the reed snapped (because of the thyroid enlargement), this indicated a pregnancy.

Hyperthyroidism and Pregnancy

Although the thyroid gland gets larger during pregnancy, its function remains the same. In other words, pregnancy does not cause either an underactive or overactive thyroid. However, hypothyroidism and hyperthyroidism may be found in pregnant and nonpregnant women alike.

The fetus' thyroid begins to take form at the end of the first trimester of pregnancy, about the tenth to twelfth week. During this time it produces small amounts of thyroid hormone. The fetal thyroid is vulnerable to antithyroid medication taken by the mother such as methimazole, propothiuracil, or radioactive iodine. If the fetal thyroid is affected by these medications, the developing baby may be born hypothyroid, with not enough thyroid hormone produced to sustain normal development.

Lynn is a thirty-two-year-old advertising executive pregnant with her first child:

> I am two months pregnant and I have a terrible case of morning sickness. I've been vomiting so much that I am losing weight instead of gaining. My doctor said it's normal for pregnant women to throw up, but I have a history of hyperthyroidism. Could my thyroid be acting up again now that I am pregnant?

Often it is difficult to distinguish the symptoms of hyperthyroidism from those of normal pregnancy. The symptoms of both conditions may overlap. For example, feeling warm all the time, excessive sweating, emotional excitement, nervousness, vomiting, or a racing heartbeat may be common to both normal pregnancy as well as hyperthyroidism.

There are two symptoms, however, that are specific only for hyperthyroidism. A very rapid heart rate—above 100 beats per minute—and weight loss are two important traits of hyperthyroidism. If you are pregnant and are experiencing these symptoms, you should be tested for hyperthyroidism. You will need treatment to prevent the hyperthyroidism from causing problems with your pregnancy.

Your doctor should ask you questions about all of your symptoms, comparing the ones you are experiencing now during your pregnancy with the ones you might have had in the past. You should also have a careful physical examination to check your thyroid, reflexes, heart rate, blood pressure, and other important indicators. A diagnosis of hyperthyroidism should be confirmed by blood tests. These routine thyroid function tests are described in more detail in appendix I.

Another type of blood test, *thyroid-stimulating immunoglobulins*, may be elevated if you have a particular type of hyperthyroidism called Graves' disease. This test may be elevated even if you are not currently experiencing any symptoms of hyperthyroidism. It is important to follow these levels of thyroid-stimulating immunoglobulins with blood tests every few months if you are pregnant because elevated levels may have a profound effect on the newborn baby (see chapter 7).

Once the diagnosis of hyperthyroidism has been made, it is important to determine what is causing your overactive thyroid. The most common cause is Graves' disease, although *toxic nodule*, *thyroiditis*, and *toxic multinodular goiter* may also be the cause. Each of these causes has a different treatment. In the chapter on hyperthyroidism (chapter 3) we discuss how to distinguish among these various types of hyperthyroidism by performing a nuclear scan. However, this type of test cannot be used if you are pregnant because it uses radioactive materials that are taken up by the thyroid gland. Even small amounts of these radioactive substances can be taken up by the fetal thyroid as well as by your thyroid. The fetal thyroid can be destroyed by this radioactive material, resulting in an underactive thyroid gland. If unrecognized, the newborn baby may suffer from severe mental as well as physical retardation. Always tell your physician if you are pregnant or think you might be pregnant in order to avoid tests that are potentially harmful to your baby.

Instead of nuclear scans, doctors must rely on careful physical examinations in order to determine the cause of your hyperthyroidism during your pregnancy. For example, in Graves' disease (the most common cause of this illness) your thyroid will be enlarged, growing upward in the neck. Because of the increased number and size of the blood vessels in a thyroid gland affected by Graves' disease, a slight swishing sound or "bruit" may be heard by your doctor when listening to your thyroid gland with his stethoscope. This sound is actually the noise of the increased bloodflow passing through the thyroid gland.

A *toxic nodule* will appear as a single thyroid lump, with the rest of your thyroid gland being small and shrunken due to the overabundance of thyroid hormone produced by the nodule. This extra thyroid hormone produces negative feedback to the brain, shutting down the remainder of the thyroid gland and causing it to shrink or "atrophy." If you have *toxic nodular goiter* you will have more than one nodule that is overactive. Finally *thyroiditis* may cause a tender and painful enlargement of your thyroid gland that alerts your doctor to this form of hyperthyroidism.

Hyperthyroidism affects less than 1 percent of all pregnancies, but it has important consequences for both the mother and fetus. Therefore it is important to recognize and treat this illness.

Although many women with hyperthyroidism experience changes in their menstrual cycle—usually, irregular periods and lack of ovulation—these changes have not translated into infertility problems in women with only mild hyperthyroidism.

On the other hand, once a woman with hyperthyroidism becomes pregnant, there is an increased risk of miscarriage, spontaneous abortion, fetal growth retardation, premature labor and delivery, congenital malformations, and possibly pre-eclampsia. Fetal death may occur as a result of chromosomal abnormalities such as Down's syndrome. These risks are decreased in women whose hyperthyroidism is recognized early and treated appropriately.

Hyperthyroidism may affect the mother as well as the developing fetus. The most serious complication from untreated hyperthyroidism is heart disease, specifically heart failure as a result of the heart working overtime in response to the thyroid hormones stimulating the heart to beat faster and faster. Potentially, a more serious complication of untreated hyperthyroidism is called thyroid storm. Usually a stressful triggering event such as labor, cesarean section, or untreated infection can cause the hyperthyroidism to spin out of control. This excess of thyroid hormone can cause death if not diagnosed and treated promptly.

The treatment of hyperthyroidism in pregnant women is not the same as for a nonpregnant woman or for a man. Many of the treatments that are used for hyperthyroidism can be harmful to the developing fetus or can be passed to the newborn baby via the breast milk. The goal for the treatment of hyperthyroid women is twofold: to cure the mother and to protect the developing fetus.

Propothiuracil (PTU) is the most commonly used drug to treat hyperthyroidism during pregnancy. It acts in several ways, including blocking iodine from entering the thyroid cells, thus rendering them unable to produce thyroid hormone. This drug may weaken the body's immune system. This effect is important in treating Graves' disease, which is caused by abnormal antibodies (attackers) that are aimed at incorrectly stimulating the thyroid to produce an overabundance of thyroid hormone. PTU may decrease the amount of these attackers in the bloodstream and therefore control the disease. Because PTU can only act by preventing newly manufactured thyroid hormone from being created, previously formed thyroid hormone can persist in the blood circulation for as long as four to six weeks, thus taking a long time for the hyperthyroidism to be controlled.

Pregnancy is almost like an organ transplantation. Because the developing fetus contains genetic material from the father that is different from the mother's, the mother's body must create a compensatory mechanism to avoid rejecting the developing fetus. This mechanism is a form of decreased immune system, which allows the baby to grow and flourish. Because of these effects on the immune system, pregnancy itself may improve the course of the Graves' disease, resulting in a decreased amount of medication needed to control the illness. After delivery, however, the disease may flare up again as your body's immune system returns to normal, thus necessitating more medication. Therefore it is important to be followed at least on a monthly basis throughout pregnancy and the postpartum period.

Although PTU can cross the placenta to reach the fetus' bloodstream, the risk of harm to the fetus is minimal if you are placed on the lowest possible dose necessary. Without treatment, your baby is at risk for spontaneous abortion and premature delivery. The risks and benefits of each individual situation must be carefully measured whenever starting drug therapy in a pregnant woman. No long-term ill effects have been noted in intellectual development of those children born to mothers taking PTU for hyperthyroidism during their pregnancy.

Other medications commonly used to treated nonpregnant hyperthyroid people such as beta blockers (to control heart rate) and iodides (see Appendix II) cannot be used in pregnancy because they may cause problems with your placenta, growth retardation of the fetus, or underactive fetal thyroid. Therefore these drugs are only used in extreme circumstances when the mother's life is in danger or when thyroid surgery is required.

Another treatment that is commonly used for hyperthyroidism is radioactive iodine. This therapy is discussed in detail in chapter 3. This form of treatment, however, cannot be used during pregnancy because the radioactive iodine may destroy the fetal thyroid as well as the mother's thyroid gland, resulting in a hypothyroid baby. Not only is that baby at risk for intellectual and physical growth retardation, but the hypothyroidism may cause severe enlargement of the baby's thyroid gland. The gland may be so large that it interferes with normal vaginal delivery, necessitating a cesarean section.

Finally, the last treatment for hyperthyroidism is thyroid surgery. Operations are reserved for those pregnant women who cannot take antithyroid medication (for example if you have an allergic reaction to these drugs or require very high doses to control your disease). Thyroid surgery may be performed safely during pregnancy if you are properly prepared with antithyroid drugs in order to avoid "thyroid storm"—an acute worsening of hyperthyrodism resulting in high fever, rapid heart rate, and sometimes death if not recognized and treated immediately. The safest time to operate on a pregnant woman is during the second trimester because the risks of miscarriage (during the first trimester) or premature labor and delivery (third trimester) are minimized.

Even if you are take the appropriate medicine, during your pregnancy and your hyperthyroidism is successfully treated, your baby is still at risk for the development of hyperthyroidism called neonatal thyrotoxicosis. Even with proper medication or surgery, thyroid-stimulating antibodies may remain in your bloodstream and may be passed to your newborn baby. Thus, your baby must be tested (with a simple blood test) immediately after birth for a possible overactive thyroid gland.

In addition, antithyroid drugs taken by you during your pregnancy may pass through the bloodstream and placenta to your baby, thus masking your newborn baby's hyperthyroidism for seven to ten days while these medications wear off. Careful follow-up by the baby's pediatrician is essential. Although less than 2 percent of babies who are born to mothers with Graves' disease suffer from newborn hyperthyroidism, the mortality rate of this disease if not recognized and properly treated is as high as 20 percent.

Both of the commonly used antithyroid drugs, methimazole and PTU, are passed through the breast milk into your newborn baby. In high doses, these medications may block the baby's thyroid gland, causing hypothyroidism. This underactive thyroid may result in severe intellectual and growth retardation. PTU passes into the breast milk less readily than methimazole does, and therefore PTU is preferred for mothers who are breast-feeding. However, because of the risk of hypothyroidism for the baby, only mothers who are on extremely low doses of PTU should be allowed to breast-feed. The children of these mothers should be followed closely by their pediatricians. If the dose of PTU needs to be increased, the mothers should bottle feed rather than nurse their baby.

Infertility

Although there are many different causes of infertility, hypothyroidism or an underactive thyroid is considered to be one of them. If you are hypothyroid, you may not ovulate, and it may be difficult for you to become pregnant. In addition, some researchers believe that women with untreated hypothyroidism who do conceive are at increased risk for their children to be born with physical abnormalities as well as mental retardation. Spontaneous abortion and fetal death are two other potentially serious complications of untreated hypothyroidism. Diagnosing your hypothyroidism and treatment with thyroid hormone medication will cure you of your thyroid disease.

Taking thyroid hormone medication, however, will only counteract infertility if you or the father are suffering from an underactive thyroid gland. Do not take thyroid hormone medication unless your doctor has diagnosed you as having hypothyroidism and has prescribed this medication for you. Taking unnecessary medication (if you do not have hypothyroidism) could be dangerous, because if you did conceive, the overabundance of thyroid hormone medication in your bloodstream might cause miscarriage, premature labor, or other problems in carrying the pregnancy to term.

Because many of the symptoms of normal pregnancy such

as weight gain, fatigue, and swelling overlap with the symptoms of hypothyroidism, it may be difficult to make this diagnosis if you are pregnant. Standard thyroid function blood tests will make this diagnosis with certainty, allowing your doctor to provide you with successful treatment.

The treatment for hypothyroidism during pregnancy is the same as the treatment for the nonpregnant hypothyroid person, namely thyroid hormone medication. This treatment is safe for the developing baby because it cannot cross the placenta into the baby's bloodstream. Although the causes of hypothyroidism include several different types of thyroid illnesses, the treatment with thyroid hormone medication is the same.

Only tiny amounts of thyroid hormone medication are excreted in breast milk. Therefore, there is no danger to the newborn baby if you are breast-feeding. In addition, it is important to have normal thyroid function in order to produce an adequate supply of breast milk. If you have an underactive thyroid you must be treated with thyroid hormone medication in order to breast-feed successfully.

Thyroid Disease After Pregnancy

Susan is a thirty-five-year-old lawyer who just delivered her first baby.

"Since I had my baby I've been crying all the time. I fight with my husband. I can't sleep at night. I've always wanted a baby and now I have a healthy beautiful one. What's the matter with me?"

Maybe nothing is the matter with Susan. Many women experience a temporary depression or sadness after delivery due to fatigue, hormonal fluctuations, and emotional changes. However, sometimes these symptoms, if prolonged, can be due to thyroid disease.

Thyroid illnesses are frequent after childbirth and may occur up to one year after delivery. No one knows the exact incidence of thyroid problems in postpartum women, but it is estimated to occur in up to 10 percent of women after delivery.

We do know that if you have an autoimmune disease—such a diabetes, Graves' disease, premature graying of the hair, rheumatoid arthritis, or vitiligo—you are at increased risk to develop autoimmune thyroid disease (like Graves' disease, see chapter 3; or Hashimoto's thyroiditis, see chapter 2), especially after pregnancy. In addition, some forms of postpartum thyroid disease may place you at increased risk to develop this illness again with subsequent pregnancies.

Postpartum thyroid disease can be the result of an overactive thyroid, an underactive thyroid, or both. Since many of the symptoms of thyroid disease are subtle and often overlap with the postpartum experiences of healthy women, the diagnosis of thyroid disease is often not considered. You may experience anxiety, insomnia, difficulty concentrating, irritability, weight changes, or fatigue. You may be told that these symptoms are normal after delivery, and your doctor may never even suspect thyroid disease as the cause of these symptoms. In fact, postpartum thyroid dysfunction was not even recognized as a disease until about fifty years ago.

The most common cause of postpartum thyroid disease is thyroiditis, inflammation of the thyroid gland. No one understands completely why the thyroid becomes inflamed, but the most common reason is an autoimmune process.

In autoimmune disease, your body no longer recognizes a

part of itself as belonging to your body. There is confusion, so that the body thinks that your thyroid is foreign. The body then produces antibodies in order to destroy this foreign intruder. These antibodies destroy their target organ, the normal thyroid gland. When the thyroid is destroyed, thyroid hormone is leaked into the bloodstream, thus creating a hyperthyroid, or over-functioning thyroid condition. On the other hand, so much thyroid tissue can be destroyed that there is not enough thyroid hormone left and this destruction results in an underactive thyroid gland.

Within the first one to four months after delivery, the hyperthyroid or overactive phase is most common. You may have a slight enlargement of the thyroid gland and you may notice increased anxiety, restlessness, insomnia, weight loss, and difficulty concentrating.

The overactive phase is diagnosed by blood tests to measure the abnormally increased levels of thyroid hormone in the blood-stream and also sometimes the abnormal antibodies, antimicrosomal and antithyroglobulin antibodies (see Appendix I). A fine needle aspiration biopsy of the thyroid gland during this phase would reveal inflammatory cells attacking the thyroid gland.

The treatment for this hyperthyroid phase of the disease is waiting it out. If the symptoms are extreme, beta blockers may be used to slow the heart rate and decrease nervousness. Antithyroid drugs are generally not used because this phase usually lasts for a short period of time, about two to four months.

This second phase of postpartum thyroiditis is an underactive or hypothyroid period and usually occurs three to eight months postpartum. This phase can be characterized by a slight enlargement of the thyroid gland and symptoms of weight gain, fatigue, lack of energy, and often depression. In fact, many cases of so-called postpartum depression have actually been linked to postpartum thyroid disease and are readily treatable.

Hypothyroidism can be diagnosed by blood tests to document the decreased levels of thyroid hormone in the bloodstream and also the elevated levels of thyroid-stimulating hormone, which is the brain's way of telling the body that it needs more hormone production. Permanent hypothyroidism may develop especially if you have high antibody levels or a severe hypothyroid phase.

Treatment for this hypothyroid phase is with thyroid hormone medication for about six months. After this time, the medication is stopped to determine whether or not the thyroid has recovered its normal function. If so, the medication may be stopped permanently. However, in up to one-third of cases, the medication must be resumed because of permanent injury to the thyroid gland.

Graves' disease is another cause of postpartum hyperthyroidism. The long-term treatment of Graves' disease versus postpartum thyroiditis is quite different, so it is important to figure out which disease you have before starting treatment.

A twenty-four-hour radioactive iodine test will be able to tell these two conditions apart (see Appendix I). Remember that when you ingest a dose of iodine, it will be absorbed in your bloodstream and travel to your thyroid. Because the iodine given to you has radioactivity in it, a special camera can be used to take a picture of your thyroid gland. If you have Graves' disease, this iodine will be quickly concentrated in your thyroid gland, and the picture (taken twenty-four hours after you have had the iodine drink) will show an overactive thyroid gland.

If you have postpartum thyroiditis, however, the autoimmune process destroys the thyroid gland and the damaged thyroid cannot absorb the radioiodine. The result is a picture that shows a damaged thyroid gland. (Note: You cannot take radioactive iodine if you are pregnant or think you might be pregnant because this substance can be concentrated in the fetal thyroid, thus destroying it. You cannot take this medication if you are breast-feeding, because the radioactive material will be passed to your baby through the contaminated milk.)

9

Thyroid Disease and Nutrition and Lifestyles

Protection from Thyroid Cancer

One of the most commonly asked questions patients have is about how they can improve thyroid health and prevent thyroid cancer. Recent research comparing patients with and without thyroid cancer have shown that there may be a protective effect of eating a diet rich in beta-carotene and possibly even vitamins C and E. These studies were performed in patients with papillary and follicular thyroid cancer, the most common types of thyroid cancer. Vitamin C is found in citrus fruit such as grapefruit and oranges. Other fruits which are rich in Vitamin C are berries—strawberries, raspberries, and blackberries—as well as many vegetables, including red and green peppers. Vitamin E–rich foods include the green leafy and yellow vegetables and fruits such as lettuce, spinach, carrots, sweet potatoes, and apricots. On the other hand, vitamin D, folate, calcium, thiamin, or riboflavin showed no clear association with thyroid cancer risk.

Some trace minerals, such as selenium and zinc, may be necessary for normal thyroid function, but we do not know the effect of increased dietary intake of these elements has on long-term thyroid function. Therefore you should avoid high-dose supplements of these minerals.

Although diet and nutrition are popular medical topics, we know relatively little about their contribution to thyroid disease. We know the most about the relationship between iodine and thyroid disorders, because iodine deficiency is the most common nutritional inadequacy worldwide. Although iodine deficiency can lead to severe mental and physical growth retardation, it is quite easy to correct and treat. Despite this fact, iodine deficiency remains a worldwide health problem.

Iodine

Iodine is essential for the thyroid to make thyroid hormone. You get this important nutrient from food. Most iodine is found in salt water, but not in fresh water. Therefore if you live near the ocean and eat saltwater fish, you get plenty of iodine in your diet. Iodine in the soil, however, has been depleted by thousands of years of erosion and flooding. So in some countries, populations that live in the mountains or inland areas away from the sea, don't get enough iodine in their diet.

Since iodine is necessary to produce thyroid hormone, a deficiency of thyroid hormone triggers your brain to produce more thyroid-stimulating hormone in an effort to increase the production of thyroid hormone. However, since the process of making thyroid hormone cannot be completed without iodine, the thyroid-stimulating hormone has the effect of encouraging the thyroid to grow in size. This benign enlargement as a result of iodine deficiency is called endemic goiter.

If you have a normal thyroid to begin with, mild degrees of

iodine deficiency will cause a goiter to form, but there will still be adequate thyroid hormone production by the gland. If you are exposed to severe iodine deficiency in your diet or if you already have thyroid disease, the result may be both a goiter as well as hypothyroidism (an underactive thyroid).

Children, especially infants, are much more susceptible to the effects of iodine deficiency than are adults. If a child is severely iodine deficient he will suffer extreme growth impediments, always remaining short and never achieving his full height potential. Irreversible brain damage may occur, with poor intellectual development as well as partial or complete deafness. Pregnant women who are iodine deficient have a higher rate of miscarriage, and their children have a higher incidence of infant death than do women with an iodine-rich diet.

Although iodine deficiency is quite common worldwide (even in developed countries in Europe), only the United States and a handful of other countries have no evidence of iodine deficiency. Since 1917, iodine has been added to salt in order to eliminate the problem of iodine-deficient goiter in this country. The recommended daily requirement for iodine consumption is 150 mcg for adults, 90 mcg for small children, and 200 mcg for pregnant women.

In order to fulfill these daily requirements, you need to eat foods that contain iodine. In addition to salt, iodine is found in seafood, seaweed, milk, eggs, and meat. Fruits and vegetables have very low iodine, except spinach, which is iodine rich.

Many people think that if a little bit of iodine is good for you and maintains normal thyroid function and size, that a lot of iodine is even better for you. This assumption is definitely not true. Although most people who have normal thyroid glands can consume more than ten times the recommended daily allowance with no ill effect, other people who are susceptible to underlying thyroid disease may be harmed by large quantities of iodine in the diet. If you purposely eat huge quantities of iodine, such as is found in seaweed kelp tablets, your thyroid hormone production may be blocked, also causing goiter and an underactive thyroid.

Additionally, if you already have an overactive thyroid, hyperthyroidism, you should avoid these excessive amounts of iodine in your diet because it may cause your hyperthyroidism to worsen (called the "Jod-Basedow" phenomenon).

Iodine is absorbed in the digestive system. Therefore if you have chronic diarrhea or other intestinal diseases with poor absorption, you may not be able to absorb dietary iodine. If you have this problem, your doctor will want to check your thyroid function blood tests once a year to make sure your thyroid is functioning normally.

Worldwide efforts to provide dietary supplements of iodine have been implemented during this century. Iodine can be added to salt or water supplies. In addition, it can be mixed with vegetable oil and given as a shot in your muscle that will provide adequate iodine supplies for up to three years.

Goitrogens

Some foods can cause a goiter by blocking the effects of thyroid hormone. These foods are called goitrogens and include cruciferous vegetables such as cabbage and broccoli. If these foods are cooked, however, the goitrogens are inactivated and their effects on the thyroid are blocked. Other goitrogens include cyanoglucosides, which are found in cassava (a tropical plant), maize, bamboo shoots, sweet potatoes, and lima beans. Additionally, these goitrogens may have their most harmful effect on people who live in iodine-deficient areas.

Vitamins

In addition to iodine deficiency, thyroid problems are generally more severe in people with vitamin A deficiencies. Therefore, you should eat a healthy supply of vitamin A–rich foods such as low-fat dairy products, fortified cereals, deep yellow or orange vegetables (carrots), and dark green vegetables. It is best to get your vitamin A supply from the foods listed above, rather than taking vitamin A supplements. Vitamin A is stored in body fat and is not released from the body for a very long time. Therefore, if you take more than the recommended daily allowance of vitamin A tablets, the extra vitamin A will be stored in your body fat in excessive amounts and can actually poison you. Always read your vitamin labels to make sure you are not taking too much.

Iron deficiency may also worsen the thyroid disease caused by iodine deficiency. Again, it is best to get your iron from natural food sources. Iron rich foods include beef; liver; dark green leafy vegetables such as spinach and kale; legumes like peas, lentils, and lima beans; as well as soybeans and soy products.

Caffeine

If you are hyperthyroid, you should avoid foods and drinks that contain caffeine, such as coffee, tea, chocolate, and soda. These foods contain a compound called methyl xanthene that acts as a diuretic (meaning it causes you to urinate frequently and in large amounts). Dehydration may result, thereby worsening the signs and symptoms of hyperthyroidism.

Further, the stimulating effects of caffeine may affect your heart, also worsening problems with a rapid and/or irregular heartbeat. Because caffeine also speeds up the intestine, you may also have diarrhea. Frequent bowel movements or bloating may also be more severe.

Alcohol

If you are hypothyroid, you should avoid alcohol, which may worsen the symptoms of fatigue and difficulty concentrating.

Cigarette Smoking

Although we do not fully understand the exact mechanism of action between cigarette smoking and thyroid function, we do know that tobacco has a negative impact on the thyroid gland. Additionally, there are more smokers with Graves' disease and the associated eye problems, called ophthalmopathy, than would be expected in the general population.

If you have hypothyroidism, you may be making your symptoms worse by smoking. In addition, if you have hyperthyroidism, you should also avoid nicotine. This substance, found in cigarettes, chewing tobacco, and cigars can stimulate your body's metabolism. Since your body is already overstimulated because of the excess of thyroid hormone, nicotine could potentially worsen the situation.

Alternative Medicine

Complementary care treatments such as acupuncture, yoga, and meditation may provide you with a positive attitude and improve some of the troubling symptoms of your hyperthyroidism such as insomnia and nervousness, but these treatments should never be used to provide definitive treatment. From a scientific standpoint, no one has ever shown that these treatments can cure thyroid disease.

Appendix I
Diagnostic Studies

Currently, we have many new, exciting and easy ways to diagnose thyroid disease. These range from simple blood tests to sophisticated X-ray tests or specialized biopsies.

Blood Tests

Thyroid Function Tests
Throughout this book we commonly refer to a set of standard blood tests called thyroid function tests. This routine panel (one tube of blood) is usually composed of four parts, the serum total thyroxine, the triiodothyronine resin uptake test, the free thyroxine index, and the serum thyrotropin-stimulating hormone (TSH). Because of cost, not all laboratories perform each of these tests routinely. Rather, many doctors start off by ordering the TSH test and if this is abnormal, they perform the additional tests on your stored blood sample (so you don't have to have your blood drawn a second time) to provide more information.

SERUM TOTAL THYROXINE

The *serum total thyroxine* (abbreviated as the *total T4*) is a measure of the amount of thyroid hormone (T4) in your bloodstream. Remember that the thyroid makes thyroid hormone (T4), which allows the body's metabolism to function normally. This measurement includes both T4 that is circulating freely in your bloodstream as well as T4 that is bound to proteins in the blood—in other words, some of the thyroid hormone is floating in your bloodstream, like swimmers in the ocean, and other thyroid hormone is being carried by proteins in the blood, like passengers being carried on a boat. The total T4 is usually elevated in hyperthyroidism, reflecting the overabundance of thyroid hormone in your bloodstream with an overactive thyroid.

There are, however, situations in which the amount of protein that binds T4 may be elevated (when there are extra boats available to carry the passengers), therefore falsely elevating the total T4 measurement. This increase in protein is seen when you are pregnant or taking hormones such as birth control pills or estrogen. In these instances, it may be necessary to eliminate the bound T4 (passengers on the boat) from the test and focus solely on the free T4 (swimmers in the ocean) in order to determine if you are hyperthyroid or not. In these circumstances, an additional blood test called the *serum free thyroxine index* (or *free T4*) may be ordered. An elevated free T4 test is proof positive of hyperthyroidism.

TRIIODOTHYRONINE RESIN UPTAKE

Sometimes the *free T4* test may not be available (it is a sophisticated and expensive test that is not widely available at all laboratories) and the *triiodothyronine resin uptake* test (*T3 resin uptake*) may be used to indirectly measure the level of these additional proteins (boats) in your bloodstream. The most important of these proteins is called *thyroid binding globulin* or *TBG*. Again, there may be increased levels of TBG if you are pregnant. In this instance, where there is extra TBG in the bloodstream, the total T4 may be increased, while the T3 resin uptake may be decreased. If the total T4 and T3 resin uptake are both decreased, there is not enough thyroid hormone in your body; in other words, you are hypothyroid. In hyperthyroidism, however, the exact opposite is true: both your total T4 as well as your T3 resin uptake are elevated.

Free Thyroxine Index

The *free thyroxine index* (*FTI*) is not a measured laboratory test, rather it is a calculation performed by the laboratory computer. It multiplies the total T4 and T3 resin uptake in order to provide similar information to the free T4 test. The free T4 test is still more accurate than the combined use of the total T4 and T3 resin uptake tests, but remember, the free T4 test is not always available, and this calculation can be used as a rough estimate.

Serum Thyrotropin-Stimulating Hormone

The *serum thyrotropin-stimulating hormone* (*TSH*) assay is the most sensitive indicator of an underactive or overactive thyroid, and for this reason is often the first and only test ordered by your doctor. TSH is produced by the brain in order to stimulate the thyroid to produce thyroid hormone. Too much TSH in the bloodstream indicates that the brain is trying to excite your thyroid to produce more hormone. In other words, not enough thyroid hormone is present in the blood, causing the brain to produce abnormally high levels of its TSH. This condition is known as hypothyroidism.

Low levels of TSH in your bloodstream show that you have hyperthyroidism. The extra thyroid hormone produced by your overactive thyroid gland is telling your brain to turn off its production of TSH.

In the past, our ability to measure TSH directly was limited. However with the invention of an ultrasensitive (sometimes called third-generation) test, the accuracy of the TSH assay has increased dramatically.

Serum Total T3

Another blood test that is sometimes included in this panel is called *serum total T3*. Remember that like T4, T3 is a form of thyroid hormone that is mostly produced by the conversion of T4 to T3 in your bloodstream. There are some instances of hyperthyroidism, especially in the elderly, where it is the level of T3 and not T4 that is increased. Therefore if your TSH level is low indicating hyperthyroidism, but your level of T4 is not elevated, your serum total T3 should be checked in order to eliminate this possibility of T3 hyperthyroidism.

Note: Remember that the explanation of blood tests presented here is just an overview. Many medications such as estrogen, birth control pills, or other illnesses such as liver disease or hepatitis, may interfere with these measurements. It is always important to tell your doctor what medications you are taking as well as your complete medical history, in order to ensure that these tests are interpreted correctly. In addition, there are other relatively rare forms of hypothyroidism and hyperthyroidism that may produce different results than those discussed here. A skilled thyroid physician will be able to make these diagnoses by carefully ordering additional, nonroutine tests and interpreting them knowledgeably.

Thyroglobulin

Thyroglobulin is a special substance (protein) produced by the thyroid that is essential for the production of thyroid hormone. Everyone who has a normal thyroid will have a normally low level of thyroglobulin in the bloodstream. If the thyroid is injured in some way, due to inflammation (thyroiditis) for example, thyroglobulin will leak into the bloodstream. Your thyroglobulin blood test will be elevated in these circumstances. If your thyroid is removed or destroyed completely, by surgery or radioiodine treatment for example, there should be no detectable levels of thyroglobulin in your bloodstream.

Certain common types of thyroid cancer such as papillary thyroid cancer and follicular thyroid cancer may produce thyroglobulin. This test is useful after surgery for thyroid cancer because an elevated thyroglobulin test after complete removal of the thyroid gland may indicate recurrent or metastatic disease. Therefore, this blood test is routinely used to follow you after your surgery for thyroid cancer. Your doctor will probably order this test every six months for the first two years after your surgery and then once a year after that for the rest of your life. If your test is elevated, your doctor will want to order a radioactive iodine scan (see below) to see if the cancer has recurred. If so, there are many good ways to treat this cancer (see chapter 5).

Finally the thyroglobulin blood test may be useful in identifying people who are abusing their thyroid hormone medication and taking an excess number of pills. These people will appear hyperthyroid, as patients with Graves' disease do. However, thyroglobulin measurements will only be elevated in people with Graves' disease and not in those who are taking too much thyroid hormone medication. Remember, it is dangerous to abuse your thyroid hormone medication—it could lead to a heart attack. Always follow your doctor's advice.

Thyroid Antibodies

There are three main types of *thyroid antibodies* that can be routinely tested in your blood sample: *antimicrosomal antibodies*, *anti-thyroglobulin antibodies*, and *thyroid-stimulating immunoglobulins*.

In general, antimicrosomal antibodies are a more sensitive measure of thyroid disease than anti-thyroglobulin antibodies are and for this reason many doctors order only the antimicrosomal antibody test. This test is elevated in autoimmune diseases where there is inflammation of the thyroid gland such as Hashimoto's thyroiditis. Over 80 percent of people with Hashimoto's thyroiditis will have elevated levels of antimicrosomal antibodies in their bloodstream. These antibodies are routinely used to help make the diagnosis of Hashimoto's thyroiditis.

If you have Graves' disease, another form of autoimmune thyroid disease, you may also have elevations of your antimicrosomal antibodies; however, this test is not routinely used to make the diagnosis of Graves' disease. The diagnosis of Graves' disease is discussed in detail in chapter 3, and includes routine thyroid function tests to confirm an overactive thyroid, coupled with a nuclear scan to eliminate other causes of hyperthyroidism.

Thyroid-stimulating immunoglobulins (*TSI*) are specific to Graves' disease, although they are not routinely used for diagnostic purposes because this laboratory value does not alter the treatment of the disease (and it is expensive). TSI measurements are used during pregnancy however, because if you have or have had Graves' disease and have an elevated TSI test, your newborn baby is at risk for developing hyperthyroidism because TSI may cross the placenta via your bloodstream and overexcite the developing fetal thyroid. If your TSI level is elevated during your pregnancy, you obstetrician will want to follow your baby closely to check for signs of an overactive thyroid, such as a rapid fetal heart rate.

Sometimes, if you have Graves' disease, you may not have any of the usual signs and symptoms of hyperthyroidism (such as nervousness, sweating, insomnia, and a rapid heartbeat). Instead you may only have problems with your eyes—bulging, staring eyes, called Graves' orbitopathy (see chapter 3). If Graves' orbitopathy is the only symptom of the disease that you are experiencing (called euthyroid Graves' disease), your thyroid function blood tests and nuclear scans will be normal. The only way to make the diagnosis of Graves' disease in this situation is through the measurement of an elevated TSI. Treatment for euthyroid Graves' disease is directed at improving your eye symptoms (see chapter 3).

Calcitonin

The *calcitonin* blood test may be used to detect medullary thyroid cancer, a relatively rare form of thyroid cancer. Calcitonin is a substance secreted by the C-cells of the thyroid gland (these are the cells in between the main type of thyroid cell, called the follicular cells). No one knows the exact role of these C-cells, except to make calcitonin, and no one knows the exact role of calcitonin in your body. We do know, however, that calcitonin is a very good test to detect medullary thyroid cancer, which is a cancer of the C-cells.

This test may be used if your doctor finds a lump in your

thyroid in order to diagnose a medullary cancer. It may also be used after thyroid surgery has been performed to determine cancer recurrence or metastatic disease. Finally, it may be a useful screening test to detect thyroid abnormalities in family members, because some forms of medullary thyroid cancer run in families. This test may help to detect the disease early and provide for prompt surgical treatment (see also chapter 5).

Carcinoembryonic Antigen

Carcinoembryonic antigen determination (CEA) is a tumor marker found in your blood and is used for detecting medullary thyroid cancer. CEA levels may be elevated if you have medullary thyroid cancer. After surgery for this type of cancer, CEA levels may be followed every year. They should return to normal levels after curative surgery. A rise in CEA after operation could signal a recurrence of the disease.

Although CEA is not specific to medullary thyroid cancer (it is also used to follow other types of cancers, such as colon cancer), it is helpful in long term follow-up if you have been treated for medullary thyroid cancer.

Thyroglobulin RT-PCR

This is a new and experimental blood test developed to try to provide early detection and treatment for metastatic thyroid cancer. *RT-PCR* stands for *reverse transcriptase polymerase chain reaction*, which is a modern technology used to detect minuscule amounts of genetic material. The test is performed on a standard blood sample looking for genetic material specific for the protein thyroglobulin (remember that this protein is produced only be thyroid cells). If the genetic material is detected, this is evidence that thyroid cells are circulating in your bloodstream, possibly trying to spread the thyroid cancer to other places in your body, such as lungs and bone. Because this test is still being evaluated in the laboratory, it is not widely available across the country.

Imaging Tests

There are many different modalities available to image or visualize the thyroid gland, however they must be used with discrimination. A careful physical examination by a skilled doctor can often provide the exact same information as a fancy and expensive test. Be sure you know why your doctor has ordered a particular test, what the indications are, and why it's important for you. None of these tests should be ordered in a "routine" fashion, but rather for specific indications.

Ultrasound

Ultrasound is a special sound with a pitch so high that the human ear cannot hear it. An ultrasound machine records these ultrasounds to create a two-dimensional image, in this case of the thyroid.

After placing some jellylike liquid on the front of your throat, a wand (transducer) is used to take pictures of your thyroid gland. This painless test can show the size and shape of your thyroid gland. If thyroid lumps are identified, the ultrasound machine can accurately measure them. Therefore, this is a good test to use for serial examinations in order to follow a thyroid nodule to see if it is growing or shrinking over time.

The ultrasound is also helpful in determining if a nodule is solid or fluid filled (cystic), which may impact both diagnosis and treatment. Finally the ultrasound machine is most helpful in visualizing the thyroid in people who are difficult to examine physically—for example, if you have had part or all of your thyroid removed because of a cancer, it may be difficult for your physician to examine your neck because of normal scarring that occurs after thyroid surgery. In this situation, ultrasound may better visualize the remaining thyroid tissue, while also being able to detect any new thyroid cancer. Similarly, if you are obese or have a short, muscular neck that is difficult to examine, ultrasound may be useful in determining your thyroid's size and contours. Ultrasound can also be used to perform a biopsy by guiding the needle into the center of the lump when a lump is so small that it cannot be felt.

Despite ultrasound's usefulness in identifying the thyroid shape and possible nodules, it cannot tell the difference between a cancerous nodule and a noncancerous one. Only a biopsy can tell the difference between benign and malignant thyroid disease (see below).

CT Scan

A computed tomography or *CT scan* is a specialized type of X-ray that can give an accurate picture of your thyroid as well as the surrounding structures, such as muscles, trachea (windpipe), esophagus (swallowing tube), and lymph nodes (glands). CT scans are rarely used in the routine evaluation of thyroid disease. This test is not good for detecting very small thyroid nodules, but can sometimes provide additional information if you have a large nodule.

For example, sometimes an enlarging thyroid (goiter) can develop a downward growth, pushing itself behind the breast bone. Because the breast bone (sternum) is hard and the thyroid cannot be felt behind it, it is impossible to tell how far down into your chest the thyroid may have grown. Thus, CT scan may be helpful in determining the extent of thyroid enlargement.

CT scan may also tell if the thyroid nodule or mass extends beyond the thyroid, for example invading surrounding structures such as the trachea or windpipe.

CT scan requires the use of a contrast dye, which distinguishes the area being scanned from the surrounding area. This dye is a special material that is injected into your arm through an intravenous line. Some people are violently allergic to this contrast material. In addition, because this contrast material contains iodine, a CT scan may delay further treatment with radioactive iodine for up to two months, until this iodine is eliminated from the body.

Finally, CT scan may be useful in evaluating congenital thyroid abnormalities, such as thyroglossal duct cyst or lingual thyroid (see chapter 7).

If you have thyroid cancer, CT or MRI (see below) may be helpful in determining the size and extent of the cancer and whether or not there are suspiciously enlarged lymph nodes in the area.

MRI

Magnetic resonance imaging or *MRI* is a special type of imaging study that provides similar information to the CT scan. It tells about the anatomy (size and shape) of the thyroid gland, but doesn't provide information about its function (too much thyroid hormone or too little).

Unlike CT scans, MRI does not require any contrast dye. Thus MRI is preferred if your doctor needs to have additional information about a suspicious thyroid lump. Finally, MRI has an additional advantage over CT scanning because MRI does not expose you to radiation.

MRI's big disadvantage over CT scan however, is that it requires you to undergo this test in a narrow and dark machine—and many people develop a claustrophobic reaction. (MRIs take twice as long to perform as CT scans—usually about thirty to forty-five minutes). This test is even costlier than CT scan and should only be used in limited situations where additional information regarding anatomy is required by the operating surgeon.

Nuclear Scans

Radionuclide scanning, unlike ultrasound, CT scans, and MRI provide information not only about the size and shape of the thyroid gland, but also about how well—or not well—the thyroid gland is working. These nuclear scans use a variety of agents such as technetium–99m pertechnetate or iodine–123 or iodine–131, which are given orally and taken up by your thyroid gland. Pictures of the thyroid gland are then obtained at varying time periods (hours to days) after the ingestion of these substances.

If the substance is avidly taken up by the thyroid gland, then the thyroid gland is considered to be "hot" or overactive. If these agents are not taken up well then the thyroid is called "cold" or underactive. These terms can be confusing however. For example, if you have hyperthyroidism or too much thyroid hormone, you may still have a cold scan if you have thyroiditis or inflammation of your thyroid gland. Here, your thyroid gland is destroyed by inflammation, resulting in the release of an overabundance of thyroid hormone into your bloodstream. But because the thyroid cells are destroyed, the thyroid will not take up the radionuclide because it is damaged. Thus, the thyroid will appear cold on the scan even though you have hyperthyroidism or too much thyroid hormone.

These nuclear scans may be used to look at a thyroid nodule to determine if it is hot or cold. Many practitioners routinely order a nuclear scan for their patients with thyroid nodules in order to help them decide if a nodule is cancerous or benign. Hot nodules are rarely cancerous, whereas about 10 to 20 percent of cold nodules are malignant. In other words, 80 to 90 percent of cold nodules are benign. Thus, this test has limited value in trying to determine the nature of a thyroid nodule.

1^{131} TOTAL BODY SCAN

The *radioiodine scan* (called *1^{131} total body scan*) may also be helpful in order to follow your progress if you have been treated for thyroid cancer. If you have undergone complete removal of the thyroid gland for thyroid cancer, then a radioiodine scan will not reveal any activity in the throat where the thyroid used to be located. If recurrent or metastatic disease is present, however, then there may be activity in the neck or elsewhere in the body. Identifying these early relapses is important because they may be treated with additional surgery or high doses of radioiodine, which are actively taken up by the cancer and then the radioactivity can destroy these cancer cells.

There are many problems related to the 1^{131} total body scan after you have had thyroid surgery. First, if you did not have your thyroid completely removed, the remaining normal thyroid tissue will concentrate radioiodine much more efficiently than the metastatic disease will. Therefore, leftover normal thyroid tissue will make a radioiodine scan inaccurate unless this healthy thyroid tissue is removed by surgery or higher doses of radioactive iodine are administered to destroy it.

In addition, the 1^{131} total body scan requires strict compliance with instructions in order to insure its accuracy. To obtain the best test possible, your body must be prepared to maximize the remaining normal thyroid tissue's uptake of the radioactive iodine. The way we do this preparation is to have you stop taking your thyroid hormone medication six weeks prior to the scan. In this way, your body is made to be hypothyroid with a deficiency of thyroid hormone. Once hypothyroid, the brain produces more of its thyroid-stimulating hormone in an attempt to increase thyroid hormone levels in the bloodstream. This increase in thyroid-stimulating hormone causes the most efficient concentrating of iodine by thyroid tissue because it needs the iodine to make more thyroid hormone.

Once you stop taking your thyroid hormone medication, you begin to experience the symptoms of hypothyroidism, including fatigue, difficulty concentrating, weight gain, and sometimes depression. The elderly are often most bothered by these symptoms, which can be quite disabling. In an effort to decrease the amount of time that you must be hypothyroid, we sometimes add a short-acting form of thyroid hormone called T3 (the most common brand name is called Cytomel), once you stop taking the long acting form of the medication (T4). The T4 or levothyroxine is stopped six weeks prior to the scan so that it may be eliminated from the bloodstream. At that time, T3 is started and is continued until two weeks prior to the scan. It takes two weeks for this form of thyroid hormone to be eliminated. Thus, the period of time when you are the most hypothyroid is shortened to just two weeks.

There have been some recent reports of a new drug, a pharmaceutical version of thyroid-stimulating hormone that can be given to you prior to radioiodine scanning. This drug artificially elevates the level of thyroid-stimulating hormone in the bloodstream, therefore you do not need to stop taking your thyroid hormone medication in order to achieve this effect prior to

scanning. Sometimes this method of preparing for the radioiodine scanning does not appear to be as good as the old-fashioned
way described above. In other words, the synthetic TSH may
miss some people who have metastatic thyroid cancer that
could be detected using the standard way to prepare for this
test. Ask your doctor if you are a candidate to use this new
medium.

The other important point about preparing for radioiodine
scanning is that you must avoid iodine in your diet at least one
week prior to the test. If you consume a high iodine diet prior
to this test, the radioactive iodine is not taken up as efficiently
by the thyroid because it is already saturated with the iodine
consumed in the diet. Two common sources of high iodine are
vitamins that contain iodine and shellfish. Always check medication labels thoroughly to avoid taking iodine that may be
included in standard multivitamin preparations. Second, saltwater fish and shellfish also contain high levels of iodine and
should be avoided.

Any salty foods (remember most salt in this country has
been fortified with iodine—see chapter 9) should also be eliminated. These salty foods include canned goods, cold cuts, pizza,
potato chips, pretzels, and Chinese foods. Always check the
label to see if a particular food contains large amounts of salt or
iodine.

Additionally, radioiodine scans performed after thyroid
surgery use a type of radioactive iodine called 1^{131}. In addition
to all the special preparations prior to the scan, there are also a
whole list of precautions to follow after this type of thyroid
scan. Although only a small amount of radioactivity is involved
with this scan, it is still important to follow these simple precautions in order to minimize radiation exposure to your family

members and friends. Since the radioactivity is excreted through all bodily fluids—urine, feces, sweat, and saliva (although mostly through the urine) it is essential to isolate these fluids. After you've had your 1^{131} scan, you should:

1. Always wash your hands with soap and water after you use the bathroom. Dry your hands thoroughly with a towel that only you are using.
2. Separate all towels, washcloths, and bed linen. Wash all of these items separately from the family wash.
3. In order to dilute the amount of radiation in urine and feces, always flush the toilet at least two or three times after using the bathroom.
4. Wash the bathroom sink, shower, bathtub, and bidet after each use.
5. Separate your plates, silverware, and drinking cups. Better yet, use paper plates and plastic cutlery, so you won't have to wash your dishes separately from the rest of the family.
6. If you are cooking for the family, remember not to taste any of the food with a utensil that will be used in cooking or communally. Once a utensil touches the saliva in your mouth it is considered to be contaminated and must be washed separately.
7. Sleep in a separate bed from your partner. Avoid open mouth kissing and sexual intercourse.
8. Radiation exposure is directly related to the amount of time you spend with another person as well as how intimate and close your contact is with them. Avoid prolonged intimate physical contact with babies, children, and pregnant women. You

may perform all essential duties such as changing diapers, if no one else is available to help you. Wash your hands before and after these tasks.

9. In order to flush out the radiation faster, keep yourself well hydrated (preferably with water) so that the radioactive iodine will be passed out of your body through your urine.

These precautions should be followed for three days after the 1^{131} test. After this period of time, the radiation exposure to other people is negligible and you do not need to follow any additional precautions.

SESTAMIBI SCAN

Sestamibi scanning is a newer form of nuclear scanning that uses a special radio-labeled tracer called sestamibi to identify tumors that have a lot of blood vessels in them. Because some forms of thyroid cancer metastases have many blood vessels, this test is particularly useful for identifying follicular thyroid cancer metastases to the bone and lung.

Additionally, it has a special advantage over conventional radioiodine scanning routinely used to identify thyroid cancer metastases: sestamibi scanning does not require you to stop taking your thyroid hormone medication. You also do not need to follow the list of precautions (above) after having a Sestamibi scan.

In the future, we hope that sestamibi scanning will allow us to identify which patients have metastatic thyroid cancer and are candidates for high dose radioiodine treatment.

Finally, some relatively rare thyroid cancers, such as Hurthle cell cancer (an unusual variant of follicular thyroid cancer) do not light up with radioactive iodine, but they can be seen with the Sestamibi scan. Therefore this test can be useful in the diagnosis and early treatment of these metastases.

Chest X-Ray

A routine *chest X-ray* is not a very good screening test to examine the thyroid. Although very large thyroid masses may push the trachea (windpipe) to one side because of the bulk of the thyroid gland, this tracheal shift is not specific to a thyroid mass and other types of diseases must be considered, such as lung problems.

Biopsies

All of these imaging studies, including ultrasound and CT scan, show only a picture of the thyroid and cannot tell the difference between cancer and noncancer. These tests may suggest a benign or malignant process, but they are not conclusive. It's like looking at a photograph of a delicious-looking piece of chocolate cake. It may have beautiful decorative icing and lots of layers, but looking at a photograph can't tell you if that cake actually tastes delicious—only a bite, or in the case of thyroid disease, a biopsy, can give you that information. There are two types of biopsies: *fine needle aspiration biopsy* and *coarse needle biopsy*.

Fine Needle Aspiration Biopsy

The most common type of thyroid biopsy is the fine needle aspiration biopsy. This test is relatively quick and painless. The needle used to perform the biopsy is actually much smaller than the needle that is used to draw blood from your arm for routine blood tests.

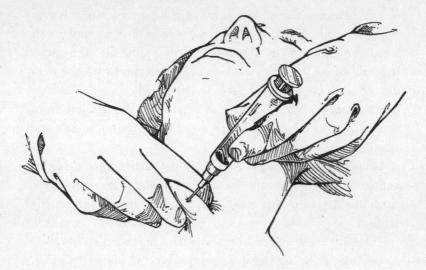

Needle Biopsy of Thyroid

The test is performed while you are lying down with your neck extended backwards. Usually a small pillow is placed underneath your shoulder blades for comfort. Your doctor may or may not use a small amount of numbing medicine before the biopsy, depending on your preference (the numbing medicine burns about as much as the biopsy needle pinches). A small needle attached to a syringe is placed into the thyroid nodule and a few cells are removed or aspirated, which are then spread on a microscope slide to be examined by the pathologist.

This test is more than 90 percent accurate in diagnosing the most common form of thyroid cancer, papillary thyroid cancer, but it is much less accurate for other forms of thyroid cancer. Often this test cannot distinguish between goiter (a benign condition), and follicular neoplasm (a premalignant or cancerous lump).

In addition, there may be a sampling error involved with using this technique. For example, if you look at an apple with a bruise on one side and randomly put a needle into the apple, it would be easy to miss the area of bruising and stick the needle only into normal portions of the apple. The same holds true of a thyroid nodule. Thus, it may be necessary to sample from several areas of a large nodule in order to try to minimize these sampling errors.

Finally, blood may interfere with the microscopic determination of a diagnosis; thus if the thyroid nodule contains many small blood vessels, this blood may produce an uninterpretable artifact.

Despite these minor limitations, the fine needle aspiration biopsy is an easy, inexpensive, and good technique in the initial diagnosis of thyroid nodules.

Coarse Needle Biopsy

A coarse needle biopsy is similar to a fine needle aspiration biopsy, but it involves the use of a much larger needle. For this reason, it can only be used by physicians experienced in this technique.

You are positioned in the same way as for a fine needle aspiration biopsy. Numbing medicine is used for the skin in the front of the throat and then a very small knife is used to make a tiny knick in the skin, which allows the physician to insert the large needle. During the biopsy procedure, you may experience some pressure in your neck, but you do not feel sharp pain. Sometimes the biopsy makes you feel like you need to cough or have a little tickle in the back of your throat.

The coarse needle biopsy removes a thin sliver of thyroid tissue, rather than just a few cells. Having an actual piece of the thyroid tissue may help the pathologist determine the architecture of the thyroid nodule and thus make a more accurate diagnosis.

Complications may occur with this type of biopsy, although they are relatively rare. The most common complication is bleeding, which occurs in less than 1 percent of all biopsies. Because the thyroid tissue may have many blood vessels within and surrounding it, using a coarse needle may cause hemorrhage, which would require an operation to remove the bleeding thyroid gland.

Other Tests

Flexible Laryngoscopy

This test is occasionally performed in order to evaluate the vocal cords. Remember that some people with thyroid disease have voice changes as a result of the thyroid cancer invading the nerves that enervate the vocal cords. Thus, one of the first detected symptoms of thyroid cancer may be a voice change.

A *flexible laryngoscope* is a small narrow telescope that is inserted into your nose (after applying lubricating jelly) down the back of your throat, and positioned just above your voice box. While watching the vocal cords through this instrument, your physician will ask you to make various sounds and observe motion of your vocal cords to see if they are paralyzed or functioning improperly.

Appendix II
Thyroid Medications

There are three main thyroid medications that may be prescribed for thyroid disease. By far the most common thyroid medication is *levothyroxine*, which is a form of thyroid hormone. Levothyroxine is sometimes referred to as T4 (see the introduction). Another form of thyroid hormone is *triiodothyronine*, or T3, which is usually prescribed for a few weeks before a radioiodine scan. *Methimazole* and *propothiouracil* are two antithyroid drugs that are used for treating hyperthyroidism. Finally, *propranolol* is a heart-rate lowering drug sometimes given for hyperthyroidism. Each of these five medications will be discussed in detail in this chapter.

Levothyroxine

Levothyroxine, thyroid hormone, is one of the top one hundred most-prescribed medications in this country. Thyroid hormone may be used for several situations, including if you have an underactive thyroid or a thyroid nodule or if you have thyroid cancer. For the first situation, if you have an underactive thyroid or hypothyroidism, thyroid hormone medication is needed to replace your own low or absent levels of thyroid hormone. For example, if you have had a thyroid operation and have had your thyroid completely removed, you are dependent on the thyroid hormone medication in order to have enough thyroid hormone in the bloodstream to live and function properly.

In the second situation, if you have a lump or nodule in the thyroid, your physician may try to shrink the nodule by giving you thyroid hormone therapy (see also chapter 4). In this situation, your brain is made to think that there is enough thyroid hormone in your bloodstream (because of the thyroid hormone medication) and your brain does not release thyroid-stimulating hormone. Without this stimulating hormone, the thyroid shuts down and shrinks. Hopefully, the nodule will also shrink. If the nodule is cancerous, however, it will usually continue to grow despite the thyroid hormone medication. A growing nodule is a reason to perform thyroid surgery in order to rule out thyroid cancer.

Lastly, if you have had thyroid surgery for thyroid cancer, your doctor will want to keep you on thyroid hormone therapy for the rest of your life. In this instance, your brain is again led to believe that there is enough thyroid hormone in the bloodstream. Thus, it does not release the thyroid-stimulating hormone. It is important to block thyroid-stimulating hormone because this hormone can stimulate thyroid cancer, causing it to grow and potentially spread.

One hundred years ago, there were very few options as to what type of thyroid hormone medication to take and how to take it. The recommendation for all people with hypothyroidism was to eat a sheep's thyroid gland once a week. To make this treatment more palatable it was suggested that the person fry it and serve with current jelly.

Later, dried or desiccated thyroid powder or tablets were obtained from animal thyroid tissue and were widely prescribed. The problem with this type of thyroid hormone preparation is that it actually contains two different types of thyroid hormone, T3 and T4. In the body, T4 is naturally converted to its active form, T3. In addition, T4 is much longer acting than T3. So when both T3 and T4 are given together, there are abnormally high peaks of T3 blood levels throughout the day, rather than a steady state of normal thyroid hormone, which is more desirable. For this reason, and because the animal preparations are highly variable and difficult to standardize, these desiccated thyroid hormones are rarely prescribed today.

Currently we have available individual, standardized, synthetic preparations of T3 and T4. For T3 preparations, it is necessary to take them two or three times during the day, because they are shorter acting than T4, thus resulting in abnormal peaks and low points of the body hormone levels throughout the day. Therefore synthetic T4, also known as levothyroxine, has replaced most other forms of thyroid hormone therapy because it is well standardized as well as being a once-a-day medication.

Thyroid hormone (levothyroxine) is generally available as a brand name as well as in many generic varieties. Recent studies have shown that the two types of T4, brand name and generic, are comparable. Many experts, however, still have their doubts. In general, try to stick to one preparation without switching brand names or different types of generic hormone. The most common brand names are Synthroid, Levothyroid, and Levoxyl. The brand-name medication costs approximately $10 to $20 for a three-month supply, while the generic forms can be as low as $3. If you switch pharmacies, ask for the same tablets you had been taking. If you are unable to continue taking the same form, notify your doctor so he can order blood tests to make sure you are taking the correct dosage.

The standard brand names of levothyroxine are color coded so that white is 50 mcg, yellow is 100 mcg, blue is 150 mcg, pink is 200 mcg, and green is 300 mcg. These color codes are often confusing, because the intermediate doses often overlap with these standard ones—for example, 75 mcg is lavender, a shade very close to the pale blue color of the 150 mcg tablet. Thus it is important to check your prescription with both your doctor and pharmacist in order to ensure that you are getting the correct dose.

The usual dose of levothyroxine is estimated based on your weight. So, for example, if you weigh 125 pounds, your estimated dose will be about 125 mcg. The usual starting dose of levothyroxine is 50 mcg per day with increases of 25 mcg every three to four weeks until you reach your estimated dose. Once you reach that dose, you need to have a blood test to make sure that this estimated dose is really the right dose for you. Because the medication is long-acting, it takes several weeks for the full effects of a dose change to be recognized. Therefore, frequent blood tests (more than every four to six weeks) are of little value.

With each dose change, blood tests (thyroid function tests) must be obtained, approximately four to six weeks after the adjustment in order to see the effect of the medication. Once you've reach your correct dose, you usually only need to have this blood test once a year. However, as you age and gain or lose weight, become pregnant, go through menopause, or take additional medications, your dose of thyroid hormone may need to be checked more frequently.

If you forget to take a dose of your medication and then remember it later in the day, go ahead and take the medication. But, if you do not remember the missed dose until the following day, do not take a double dosage, just take your usual pill as prescribed.

There have never been any reported cases of an allergic reaction to levothyroxine. However, some patients may be allergic to the dyes or fillers used to make the tablet. If this happens, your doctor will want you to change brand names.

Levothyroxine causes increased work for the heart by speeding up your metabolism. If you have heart disease, such as chest pain (angina), high blood pressure, history of a heart attack, or irregular heart rhythm, you should be monitored closely for side effects of too much medication. These side effects include chest pain, increased pulse rate, palpitations, excessive sweating, and nervousness. Any of these symptoms should be reported to your doctor immediately. If you have heart disease, you should be started on an extra low dose of thyroid hormone and be advanced more slowly, under your doctor's supervision.

Levothyroxine may interact with other medications, such as blood thinners (anticoagulants), diabetes medication, anti-ulcer medications, hormones/birth control pills, narcotic pain medication, and medicine taken to reduce high cholesterol levels. Check with your doctor if you are taking one of the above medications. For example, cholestyramine, which is a medication taken to reduce high cholesterol levels in the blood, can bind to levothyroxine and inactivate it. Thus, at least a four- to five-hour interval is recommended between taking these two medications in order to avoid this binding effect. Similarly, it is important to let your doctor know if you are taking hormones such as estrogen or birth control pills, medications or foods containing high levels of iodide (like kelp tablets), or iron or aspirin products because these medications interfere with the thyroid function blood tests obtained to monitor the dose of levothyroxine.

Finally, check with your doctor if you have intestinal problems, such as malabsorption, or if you have had intestinal surgery for obesity, because you may have trouble absorbing levothyroxine and may require higher doses.

It is always best to take your thyroid hormone medication on an empty stomach in the morning. Avoid high fiber foods immediately after taking your medication, as these may block the absorption of thyroid hormone.

There are some people who abuse their thyroid hormone medication, taking extra doses in the hopes that the levothyroxine will help them lose weight. This is not only mistaken, but dangerous as well. Studies have confirmed that in obese people with normal thyroid glands, levothyroxine will not cause weight loss. If given in large doses to patients who do not need to take this medication, extreme side effects and even death can occur (especially when given in combination with diet pills). The bottom line is that this medication is quite safe to take if you have a medical reason to take it. However, abusing this medication in order to try to lose weight is extremely dangerous.

It is safe to take thyroid hormone medication during pregnancy, however, you should always inform your doctor. Your dose of thyroid hormone medication may need to be changed during the pregnancy, so your physician should follow you more closely (probably every two to three months).

There are a few potential side effects of levothyroxine that are important to discuss. We know that people who have over-active thyroids suffer from increased bone metabolism. All the bones in your body are constantly being broken down and rebuilt. However, if you have an increased metabolism as a result of hyperthyoidism, you will have a faster rate of bone turnover. With this increase in bone remodeling, you lose essential bone minerals, which puts you at risk for osteoporosis. Because of this fact, there has been concern that taking thyroid hormone medication, especially in high doses, may also cause osteoporosis.

If you have had a previous history of an overactive thyroid, you are at increased risk for the development of osteoporosis from taking thyroid hormone medication because you already have weakened bones due to your history of hyperthyroidism.

When bone loss has been studied in both women and men who are taking thyroid hormone medication, there is essentially no bone loss reported in premenopausal women or in men. In postmenopausal women, however, there may be significant osteoporosis, especially in those women already suffering from osteoporosis. Does this loss of bone mineral density place these women at an increased risk for broken bones? No one has been able to convincingly prove that these postmenopausal women are at increased risk for bone fracture as a result of bone de-mineralization.

However, because of these concerns, we are careful to pre-scribe the lowest possible effective dose of thyroid hormone medication, especially in postmenopausal women. If you have had a history of thyroid cancer and need high doses of thyroid hormone, we are especially careful in monitoring blood tests as well as recommending calcium supplements or estrogen ther-apy (if you are a postmenopausal woman). Other risk factors for the development of osteoporosis include a lean body weight, low calcium intake, smoking, alcohol abuse, sedentary lifestyle, never having been pregnant, as well as a family history of osteoporosis. The overall risks and benefits for each individual must be carefully assessed prior to starting thyroid hormone medication.

The other main risk associated with thyroid hormone medication is heart disease. Because thyroid hormone speeds the body's metabolism, the heart must keep up with this increased demand for energy. If you already have heart problems (including high blood pressure), these extra demands may cause a heart attack. Thyroid hormone medication at high doses may cause an increased heart rate, extra beats, or an irregular heartbeat. If you have a history of heart disease, you should take thyroid hormone medication with caution and under careful supervision of your physician.

Currently there are no data to support a link between thyroid hormone medication and breast cancer. Although it is true that many women with breast cancer also have some form of thyroid disease, both diseases, breast cancer and thyroid disease, are found in women. So far, however, there has not been a proven association between the two illnesses. Therefore, thyroid hormone medication is safe for women with breast cancer or for those women who are at increased risk for the development of breast cancer.

Triiodothyronine

Triiodothyronine, or *T3* (brand name, Cytomel), is usually used in preparing you for a radioiodine scan after your thyroid surgery. This scan is used after surgery to detect remaining thyroid tissue that has not been completely removed during the operation. It is also used to see if thyroid cancer has spread to other parts of the body. Remember that normal thyroid tissue and thyroid cancer metastases will bind iodine. During a scan, radioactive iodine is given to you orally. The iodine is then bound by the leftover thyroid tissue or thyroid cancer metastases. Because this iodine is radioactive, a special camera can take a picture of it to determine if there is leftover thyroid tissue in your neck or if your thyroid cancer has spread to other parts of your body.

In order to undergo total body radioiodine scanning you must be very hypothyroid. In other words, all thyroid hormone medication must be stopped prior to the scan. By making you deficient in thyroid hormone, the high levels of the brain's thyroid-stimulating hormone cause potential thyroid cancer metastases to better take up the radioactive iodine. These metastatic sites can then be destroyed with higher doses of radioiodine.

Because levothyroxine or T4 is long-acting, it takes about one month to wash out of the bloodstream completely. If T4 is stopped, you will eventually experience the symptoms of hypothyroidism (fatigue, weight gain, difficulty concentrating) for four weeks. But because T3 is relatively short-acting, it only takes about two weeks to wash out of the bloodstream. Thus, if you stop taking your T3 medication you will only experience these unpleasant side effects for about two weeks, instead of four.

Therefore, most practitioners prepare you for a radioiodine scan by stopping your T4 and beginning T3 about six weeks prior to the scan. After four weeks all of the T4 is washed out of the system, but you never experience the symptoms of hypothyroidism during this period because you are still taking thyroid hormone in the T3 form. Two weeks before the scan, the T3 is stopped and you become hypothyroid for a brief period just prior to the scan. If no further therapy is needed after the scan (meaning if there is no leftover thyroid tissue in the neck and no spread of thyroid cancer that would require high doses of the radioactive iodine to destroy the cancer), then you can restart your normal dose of T4 medication.

Although there haven't been any reported cases of allergies to T3, if you are taking doses that are too high, you may have the same symptoms as those listed above under levothyroxine. You should always report symptoms of chest pain, increased heart rate, palpitations, excessive sweating, or nervousness to your doctor. You may need to temporarily stop the medication or reduce its dose.

The usual dose of T3 is usually between 25 and 75 mcg per day. This dose is usually given as two pills a day. So, for example, if your dose is 50 mcg per day, you will be instructed to take 25 mcg in the morning and 25 mcg in the evening.

Methimazole

Methimazole is a common medication used for the treatment of hyperthyroidism. Remember that hyperthyroidism is caused by too much thyroid hormone in your body.

The most common brand name of methimazole is Tapazole. This drug works by blocking the formation of thyroid hormone. By blocking thyroid hormone production, your body's level of thyroid hormone will eventually drop, and your hyperthyroidism will stop. At this point, the dose of methimazole may be adjusted to allow your body to make the normal level of thyroid hormone, rather than producing too much.

The most common side effects of methimazole are minor and include skin rash, hives, stomach upset such as nausea and abdominal pain, muscle aches, headache, and dizziness.

The most serious side effect of methimazole is called agranulocytosis. This problem causes a failure in blood cell production. There are three different types of blood cells that are no longer manufactured during agranulocystosis: 1) white blood cells (which fight infection), 2) red blood cells (which carry oxygen), and 3) platelets (which help make blood clots when the body is injured). Since white blood cells are important for fighting off infection, a lack of these cells can result in an overwhelming infection called sepsis, which can be deadly. Since everyone who takes the drug is at risk to develop this very rare side effect, it is extremely important to report to your doctor any fever, sore throat, skin blisters, headache, or muscle aches that you experience while taking this medication. These symptoms may mean an early infection, which can progress rapidly within hours to days. The only treatment is to stop the methimazole immediately. Serious cases of sepsis will require hospitalization and antibiotics. Most people are cured if these symptoms are recognized and treated early.

Although there is no way to tell who will develop agranulocytosis, this rare side effect is most often seen in people over the age of forty who are taking a high dose of the medication. Therefore, it is essential to take the smallest dose possible to adequately control the symptoms of hyperthyroidism.

Another rare but potentially serious side effect of the methimazole is inflammation of the liver, called hepatitis. Symptoms of this type of reaction include right-side abdominal pain, loss of appetite, fever, and skin itching. The diagnosis can be made by simple blood tests and the treatment is to stop the medication immediately. Once the methimazole is stopped, your liver will be able to recover completely.

Methimazole may react with other medications called anti-coagulants, which are used to thin the blood and prevent clotting, prescribed for diseases such as stroke or irregular heart rhythms. If you are taking blood thinners you should have blood tests every month to determine if you are on the proper dose of anticoagulant. Additionally, even if you are not taking a blood thinner, methimazole can cause bleeding. Therefore, everyone taking this medication should have a blood test to check for problems with blood clotting.

Methimazole comes in 5 and 10 mg tablets. The starting dose for mild hyperthyroidism is 5 mg every eight hours. For moderate hyperthyroidism, the dose can be increased to 10 mg every eight hours, and in severe cases, up to 20 mg every eight hours. Remember that the incidence of serious side effects of the medication increases with increasing dosage—especially higher than 40 mg per day. Thus, it is important to have the dosage monitored closely by your physician. You should try to take the lowest dose possible. Once your hyperthyroidism has been controlled, the maintenance dose of methimazole is approximately 5 to 15 mg per day. Your doctor will want to keep you on this medicine for at least six months before stopping it to see if the hyperthyroidism has gone away completely (see chapter 3).

If you are pregnant, you should not take methimazole because it may harm your baby. This drug can block the baby's thyroid from developing normally. Without the production of adequate amounts of thyroid hormone, a baby may suffer from severe intellectual, physical, and emotional growth abnormalities. Methimazole may also cause severe enlargement of the baby's thyroid, which could interfere with a normal delivery (the baby's thyroid may be so large that the baby will not fit through the birth canal and a cesarean section will have to be performed). Rarely, methimazole may also cause a skin problem in the baby called aplasia cutis, which is a bare area of the scalp. Finally, this drug should not be taken if you are breast-feeding your baby as it may promote hypothyroidism in your child.

Propylthiouracil (PTU)

PTU is another medication commonly prescribed for people with hyperthyroidism. In some instances, it can cure hyperthyroidism completely, in others it may control the hyperthyroidism until another therapy can be used. PTU may be prescribed in order to prepare you for thyroid surgery. If your hyperthyroidism is not treated before surgery, you may have a worsening of the hyperthyroidism during or immediately after the operation, called thyroid storm. This burst of hyperthyroidism may be fatal unless recognized and treated right away.

PTU acts by blocking the production of thyroid hormone as it is made in the thyroid gland, but it does not block thyroid hormone that has already been made in the bloodstream. Because of this pre-existing thyroid hormone, it may take weeks before all of this old thyroid hormone is eliminated from the bloodstream. In other words, it make take several weeks before your symptoms of hyperthyroidism begin to improve.

Always tell your doctor if you are pregnant or think you might be pregnant while taking PTU in order to avoid problems with your baby. PTU may be given to women who are pregnant, but close monitoring is essential, because only the bare minimum dose should be administered to control the mother's disease. In this way, risk to the developing fetus is minimized. Frequent monitoring (every four to six weeks) is important because you often need less medication as your pregnancy progresses. You should not take PTU if you are breast-feeding because the drug is excreted in the breast milk and may cause an underactive thyroid in the baby.

If you are taking PTU, you should be followed closely by a physician because this drug has some rare potentially serious and life-threatening side effects. Probably the most important side effect from this medication is a complication called agranulocytosis (see also above). This is a condition where the body's ability to produce white blood cells (cells which make up the body's immune system and allow it to fight infection) are blocked. Without white blood cells, common infections that your body is usually able to handle (such as a cold) can get out of control. Thus, a sore throat, fever, head ache, rash, or body aches may be the first and only warning sign that your body's immune system is disrupted. You should report these symptoms to your practitioner immediately and have basic blood tests to determine your white blood cell count immediately.

You should have liver function blood tests while taking PTU to avoid damage to your liver. This rare side effect is called hepatitis. Symptoms of abdominal pain, loss of appetite, yellow skin or itching should be reported immediately. Stopping the medication will cure this side effect.

PTU may interact with other medications, specifically blood thinners (anticoagulants). Thus you must be followed more closely with routine blood tests if you are taking PTU and an anticoagulant to avoid blood clotting problems.

Occasionally you may experience an allergic reaction to the

PTU, usually a skin rash and some itching. Notify your doctor and stop the medication immediately.

PTU is usually taken three times per day and the dose can vary from 300–900 mg per day. The starting dose is about 100 mg three times a day. The medication is dispensed in 50 mg tablets, so this would mean taking two tablets three times a day for a total of six tablets daily. The dose is then increased as needed to control your hyperthyroidism (see chapter 3 for a discussion of how long your doctor will want you to take PTU as a treatment for hyperthyroidism).

Propranolol

Beta blockers are a class of medications designed to reduce the rapid heart rate usually associated with hyperthyroidism. One of the most common beta blockers prescribed is called *propranolol* (brand name, Inderal).

Because propranolol works by reducing the heart rate, if you already have heart problems, such as an irregular heartbeat, make sure to notify your doctor. Because some people with heart ailments rely on a normal heart rate to prevent blood from backing up in the lungs, slowing the heart rate can be quite dangerous in these patients and lead to heart failure.

If you have asthma you should not take beta blockers because this type of medication may cause an asthma attack.

Finally, if you have diabetes, you should use beta blockers only with extreme caution because the lowered heart rate may mask the symptoms of a low blood-sugar level. Thus you may not realize the warning symptoms of a dangerously low blood sugar.

Propranolol may interact with alcohol, seizure medications,

Medication	Purpose
Levothyroxine (T$_4$)	• To treat hypothyroidism • To shrink thyroid nodules
Triiodothyronine (T$_3$)	• To prepare you for an 1^{131} total body scan after thyroid surgery for thyroid cancer • Occasionally used to treat hypothyroidism
Methimazole	• To treat hyperthyroidism
Propylthiouracil (PTU)	• To treat hyperthyroidism
Propranolol	• To slow a rapid or irregular heart beat which can occur with hyperthyroidism

and ulcer medications, to name a few. Always tell your doctor what other medications you are taking before starting this drug.

There are no studies to prove that propranolol is safe in pregnant or breast-feeding women. So, always tell your doctor if there is a chance that you might be pregnant. There are some circumstances however, such a thyroid storm (an acute and often life-threatening worsening of hyperthyroidism that can occur in hyperthyroid patients who are undergoing thyroid surgery) in which the benefits of propranolol outweigh its risks.

The usual dose of propranolol is between 30 and 90 mg per day. We usually start out by giving 10 mg three times a day and increase up to 30 mg three times a day if needed. Propranolol should never be stopped abruptly because there may be a rebound effect in which the rapid heart rate is worsened. Always talk to your doctor about how to slowly taper off from this medication, rather than discontinuing it suddenly.

Index